SOCIAL WORK, PSYCHIATRY AND THE LAW

For our wives, Vivienne and Josephine

Social Work, Psychiatry and the Law

Second Edition

N.N. Pringle and P.J. Thompson

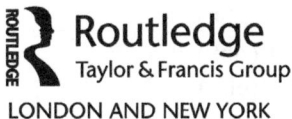

Routledge
Taylor & Francis Group

LONDON AND NEW YORK

Contents

A note about the authors

Norman Pringle, RMN, CQSW is an ASW and Mental Health Consultant.

Paul Thompson, CQSW, PGCE, MBA, UKCP Registered Psychotherapist, is an ASW External monitor/assessor and principal lecturer in social work at the University of East London.

Abbreviations

ADHD	attention deficit hyperactivity disorder
BCP	British Confederation of Psychotherapists
CCETSW	Central Council for the Education and Training of Social Workers
CKW	community keyworker
CPA	care programme approach
CPN	community psychiatric nurse
ECT	electroconvulsive therapy
MAOI	monoamine oxidase inhibitor
PACE	Police and Criminal Evidence Act 1984
RMO	Responsible Medical Officer
SDAT	Senile Dementia Alzheimer-Type
STG	Special Transitional Grant
UKCP	United Kingdom Council for Psychotherapy

Preface

Since the publication of the first edition of this book there has been a virtual transformation in the provision of mental health services. Many long-stay psychiatric asylums have been closed. Community care has been introduced. Law, policy and practice have necessitated institutional change although, at an operational level, resources and perceptions have not always kept pace with change, resulting in increased levels of stress – for service users and service providers – and sometimes public tragedy.

The revision of our book at this time is an attempt to help make sense of these changes from a social work perspective as well as contribute to the debates about what creates good professional and interprofessional practice. If we have not always provided the correct answers we hope that we have stimulated constructive debate and helped workers find some helpful thoughts and concepts.

Acknowledgements

Whilst family and friends create innumerable rich influences on any piece of written work, we would especially like to thank Kate Trew, our editor at Arena for her patience and advice in the preparation of our text, and Margaret Edwards who typed it all up into a coherent whole.

Gratitude is also owed to our clients, patients and students. Examples of work or situations presented in the text are drawn from many facets of our experience so as to ensure confidentiality whilst conveying something of the complexities of contemporary mental health practice.

Copyright note

Introduction

We have attempted, in the pages of this book, to draw together the many strands of contemporary approaches to social work, psychiatry and the law into a coherent framework. As our brief reflections on the history of mental health law and treatment in Chapters 1 and 2 show, there are a large number of factors at work in this field. Those chapters also deal with current law, policy, practice and treatment. At the time of writing, the mental health scene is still undergoing change, with concerns now being voiced about 'care in the community', the possible recognition of the need for more resources and a review of mental health services and, perhaps, legislation. At the time of writing, the debate about compulsory treatment in the community in the form of community treatment orders remains unresolved.

In the meantime, approved social workers, nurses (whether in the community or in hospitals) doctors, police, and relatives are still called upon to cope continually on a day-to-day basis, in sometimes near-impossible circumstances. Chapters 3 to 6 offer reflections and guidance for the day-to-day understanding and management of core issues in relation to a broad spectrum of service user groups.

Chapter 7 addresses the issue of cultural diversity and the need for awareness, knowledge, sensitivity but, above all, respect, when working with difference.

Chapter 8 offers information on the particular management aspects relating to substance use or addiction. Chapter 9 goes on to look at issues of dangerousness, both to self and others.

The final three chapters deal with different aspects of what might be termed professional and personal survival, including ethical dilemmas, before closing with an attempt to draw the disparate elements of the approved social worker's role into an integrated, and potentially optimistic, vision of therapeutic potential.

1 Law, policy and practice

Introduction

The history of mental health provision reflects the changing social attitudes towards the mentally ill. During the eighteenth century, when the Poor Law officers were authorised to detain paupers in madhouses under the Vagrancy Acts, the main aim was to control, contain and keep the mentally ill out of sight from the rest of the community. The mid-nineteenth century until the mid-twentieth century witnessed the emergence of the vast mental hospitals which were mainly built in the countryside at a distance from the population at large. However, in the second half of the twentieth century we began to turn away from the concept of institutional care within mental hospitals. The population of these hospitals peaked in 1954.

The introduction, in the early 1950s, of neuroleptic or antipsychotic medication had very important repercussions on the mentally ill patient's state of mind, for it calmed hallucinations and delusions and made many accessible to other forms of therapeutic interventions. In turn public opinion began to change, and mental illness – previously a taboo subject – came to be discussed like any other illness. This pharmacological revolution of the 1950s changed the face of the mental hospital, and professionals and the public were prepared to take risks. This manifested itself in more openness within the hospital and an open-door policy which began to anticipate further changes towards care in the community.

Indeed, what has emerged since the late 1950s is a policy of community care with an increase in the availability of care and treatment in the community which was reflected in many initiatives including psychiatric units attached to general district hospitals, day and residential facilities,

1

community psychiatric nurses and voluntary groups. The Mental Health Act 1983 provided the opportunity for more transformation in our thought and work. It introduced the concept of the approved social worker as well as clearly emphasising community care and putting the onus on patients' rights. Alongside the new Act we began to see the closure of the old mental hospitals which had for so long been the mainstay option for the care of the mentally ill. The process of community care which had began in the late 1950s was suddenly expected to escalate to meet these closures. Clearly, the implementation of such a vast change in policy became an overwhelming task for all concerned, not least for the patients who, in many cases, had regarded the hospitals as their homes. A great many patients had grown old in hospital and were now being asked to leave; many more were ill-prepared to cope in the outside world. The standard of community care was uneven throughout the country, as the necessary resources in terms of accommodation, staff and administration were not always in place to facilitate the complex transfer of care from hospital to community.

There were casualties, for the care that many had received was no longer available to them – certainly not in the way that they would recognise and had grown to understand. This produced, in many, a deep sense of displacement as well as, in many instances, the actuality of being homeless. More recently there have been major casualties which have led to changes in the law relating to mental health.

In this chapter we would like to share some of the practice issues of approved social work, also showing how these recent changes in the law have been incorporated into new legislation and how it has affected our work. These include the care programme approach (CPA), the supervision register and the Mental Health (Patients in the Community) Act 1995.

We will start by examining the assessment process which is the approved social worker's central duty under the Act. We will then go on to look at the main sections dealing with compulsory admissions to hospital and to the approved social worker's responsibilities and duties under the various sections of the Act.

The assessment process

Assessment

Before making an application for admission of the patient to hospital the Approved Social Worker shall interview the patient in a suitable manner and satisfy himself that detention in a hospital is in all the circumstances of the case the most appropriate way of providing the care and treatment of which the patient stands in need. (Section 13 (2) Mental Health Act 1983)

The request for an approved social worker to visit and make an assessment indicates that someone is concerned and/or is seeking immediate action. Referrals for an approved social worker to assess often come from GPs but may also come from relatives, neighbours, friends, community psychiatric nurses (CPNs) and other social workers. In fact, anyone who is concerned about someone else's mental health may contact a local authority social services department for help or advice.

In the case of the nearest relative requesting an application for admission to hospital the approved social worker has a duty under Section 13 (4) of the Mental Health Act 1983 to consider the case as soon as it is practicable and, if an application for admission to hospital is made, the reasons must be recorded in a case file to be kept by the social services department.

Whoever is requesting action, the approved social worker is called upon to be able to recognise and respond to people under stress and help them focus on the nature of the problem and what can realistically be done to ease the situation which is causing concern.

There are as many methods of assessment as there are individual social workers, and more important than following one method is perhaps to develop one's own style and feel easy with it. However, there are basic principles which can be delineated, and one strategy is given below.

An assessment strategy

Initial contact: the referral stage

Note the name and telephone number of the referrer. Ascertain their relationship to the person being referred. Find out exactly who they are concerned about and where that person lives.

An ASW referral checklist can be found later in this section. Here we help focus on crucial questions to ask and areas to cover in order to gather as much relevant information as possible on the person being referred.

Responsibility for action

Section 13 (3) of the Mental Health Act makes it clear that it is the duty of an approved social worker to make an application in respect of a patient within the area of the social services authority by whom he or she is appointed. This is a new provision of the 1983 Act, and it enables an approved social worker who is already working with a client to make an assessment for compulsory admission wherever the client happens to be. Nevertheless, it is undoubtedly good practice both to establish geographical location and make an automatic check to find out whether or not a client (or referrer) is known to the department. Much unnecessary effort on the part of all concerned can be avoided in this way.

Work with the referrer

The approved social worker needs to be able to form as complete a picture as possible of the current situation in order to judge the degree of urgency. There must be some significance in the timing of the referral and this must be discussed with the referrer and understood by the approved social worker. The latter may need to explain to the referrer the grounds for making a compulsory admission to hospital, if this is what is being requested. These are as follows:

1   The patient is suffering from a mental disorder of a nature or degree that warrants his or her detention in hospital for assessment followed by medical treatment for at least a limited period.
2   He or she ought to be detained in the interests of his or her own health or safety, or with a view to the protection of other persons (section 2 (2)).

However, even if it is apparent that there is no threat involved, the approved social worker should be responsive to all requests for help concerning someone thought to be mentally ill and at risk. If there is no urgency, the approved social worker should take the referral, as for any other client referred to the department, and arrange to see the referrer and/or client or pass them for allocation. The referrer can be encouraged to talk about what is happening to the patient at this precise moment in time.

Where is the client? Is he or she alone? What is worrying the referrer? Is the client aware of the referral and the reasons for concern? These are some of the questions that the social worker will need to ask until he or she has a satisfactory picture of the situation. He or she must be sensitive to the fact that the referrer may well be under considerable stress and, at this stage, the taking of detailed family history would not be helpful. The focus at the initial stage has to be on the degree of urgency and an assessment as to the appropriate immediate intervention needed to relieve the anxiety of the referrer and help the patient. The social worker should talk clearly and simply, be patient and listen to the referrer. If there is anything that is not clear he or she must clarify this with the referrer. The social worker will ensure that the referrer understands what action the worker is going to take, how long this is likely to take and who will be involved. The referrer or the person referred may have a communication problem, and it would be well to ascertain this in advance. Obviously, language factors are important but there are also cultural factors relating to patients from ethnic minorities – for example, the acceptability of a male doctor or social worker to a female Muslim patient. The social worker should discuss this with the referrer as it may be essential to ensure that an interpreter or other members of the family are present at the interview.

The approved social worker may wish to have available lists of local language interpreters and lists of workers for the deaf and dumb. Some knowledge of local ethnic groups may also be valuable.

Access

There may be problems about how the social worker will get to see the client. The social worker needs to clarify this with the referrer and ask if there will be someone at the house to open the door and also if there is anyone else who knows the person referred, such as a carer, CPN, neighbour, friend or relative. This information will be crucial if the client refuses to open the door and it is necessary to involve someone he or she knows and trusts.

Preparation for assessment visit

The GP must always be contacted immediately following a referral and informed of the reasons for concern. Some GPs may be reluctant to participate in a joint visit either because they have too little time or they have recently seen the patient. However, it is helpful to the client for the GP and social worker to visit together as they will be able to suggest alternatives to hospital – that is outpatients clinic, day hospital, CPN, environmental changes – if these are appropriate. If the client is known to be on the supervision register, subject to supervised discharge arrangements or CPA the nominated community keyworker should be notified. Discussion with the keyworker is vital for he or she is likely to have had the most recent professional contact with the patient, and his or her knowledge and experience of the patient will make a valuable contribution to the assessment and subsequent outcome.

Venue

The venue is usually where the patient is at the time of referral. Access arrangements will have been clarified with the referrer. However, the client may refuse to open the door or come out of the bedroom or bathroom. Under the Act:

> An Approved Social Worker of a local Social Services Authority may at all reasonable times after producing, if asked to do so, some duly authenticated document showing

that he is such a Social Worker, enter and inspect any premises (not being a hospital) in the area of that authority in which the mentally disordered patient is living, if he has reasonable cause to believe that the patient is not under proper care. (Section 115, Mental Health Act 1983)

If it is impossible to gain access, without forcing entry, to the house or room where the client is believed to be, the social worker has to obtain a warrant authorising the police to force entry and, if necessary, to remove the patient to a place of safety with a view to making an assessment and application for admission, or other alternative arrangements for treatment or care. In order to obtain a warrant the social worker has to go to a Justice of the Peace and give information, under oath, as to the reasons for concern (section 135 (1)).

A police constable is then empowered to force entry, either to enable an assessment to be made or to remove the client to a place of safety. The policeman and the approved social worker should be accompanied by a registered medical practitioner. (Section 135 is discussed at length, together with practice examples, in Chapter 11.)

Documents and information

Whatever the outcome of the assessment interview, the approved social worker should not put him or herself in the position of having to rush out looking for a telephone or collect a supply of documents. Ideally, he or she should have a documents 'kit' to take to any assessment interview. This should include:

- Application for Admission forms
- Medical Recommendation forms
- Personal Identification document
- a leaflet giving details of patient's rights if admitted to hospital
- a handbook of services available to the mentally ill and relevant application forms
- a list of community resources, voluntary animal care and religious organisations, and counselling services
- childcare information and forms for reception into care, nurseries, childminders
- details of home care services
- a fully charged mobile telephone!

Availability of a hospital bed

The approved social worker will need to know whether there is a hospital bed available if required. It is the GP's responsibility to find a hospital bed, and this can always be provisionally reserved by the GP to be available. In an emergency people normally go to hospital by ambulance, and the mentally ill person should be treated no differently. However, there will be cases in which this method of transport is not appropriate because of violence or other behaviour which is not containable in an ambulance.

Use of the police

The social worker has to consider whether or not to involve the police from the outset. This is a difficult decision and can only be decided in the light of what is known about the client's previous history and what is happening now. Past behaviour can sometimes be a good indicator of future behaviour.

Case example

A woman, diagnosed as schizophrenic, who had been in hospital several times previously begins to break her furniture and throw the pieces out of her window with considerable force, heedless of neighbours or passers by. She has a small axe and is refusing to open the door to anyone. After hours of stressful drama, it is only when the police arrive and firmly ask her to open the door does she calm down and do this. The police quickly take the axe from her. It is then possible and safe for the approved social worker and GP to assess how best to help her.

In such situations the help of the police can diminish further upset rather than escalate what is already an explosive situation.

The police can be alerted to a worrying situation so that, if necessary, they can send someone along quickly. Approved social workers may be able to build up a relationship with the local police, which can save time and energy when a crisis necessitating police intervention occurs. Most local authorities have worked out a policy with the local police about good practice in mental health situations including the use of section 136.

The assessment interview

Prior to the assessment interview the approved social worker may need to work out with the police a strategy to make the situation safe. The approved social worker will also need to discuss with other professionals how the interview should be managed and the ground that needs to be covered.

Assessment interviews with the aim of deciding whether compulsory admission is necessary are often fraught. The approved social worker cannot know what he or she might encounter, and the unexpected is always a possibility. The situation is often charged with anxiety and violence and there will be pressure on the social worker from relatives, doctor, police or neighbours to 'do something'. This usually means disposing of the 'problem' quickly.

It is worth remembering that, by the time the situation has reached the point of calling for an assessment for hospital admission, there have probably been days, or weeks, of frightening behaviour and continual stress for all involved. Now the problem can no longer be tolerated and action is being demanded. Often the social worker will be going in 'cold' without having met any of the people involved in the crisis, including other professionals.

Structure

The approved social worker should introduce him or herself and outline his or her role and the purpose of the assessment. He or she should also ask other professionals to introduce themselves and then explain their roles.

A structured approach to an assessment interview can help in that it brings a sense of order and clarity and enables those present to feel contained and held. When people are under stress they may not hear what is being said, or they may easily misunderstand and become angry or defensive. The social worker should be conscious of this throughout the interview and try to reduce tension by speaking simply, making sure that everyone understands what is being said and taking an unhurried but firm approach. All social workers will, of course, have their own individual style of working.

However, a basic principle is to try to talk to the client and the family, as adult to adult, without denying the emotions they may be experiencing, and help them talk to each other.

When people are in a disturbed, emotional state they sometimes find it difficult to function as adults, and they feel powerless. The assessment interview is a crisis and could be a turning-point both for the client and the family. It is therefore important to involve them as actively as possible in the assessment by asking them to talk to each other – for example, 'Can you tell your husband what it is that is upsetting you?' 'Your wife tells me that she thinks you need to go into hospital. Could you perhaps tell her, and all of us, what you think about that?' Often when people feel desperate and at the end of their tether they feel that they no longer have the strength to solve the problem. They may perceive the social worker as having great power, far beyond that of admitting someone to hospital for assessment, as if perhaps hoping for a miraculous resolution to a difficult problem.

Case example

The husband of an apparently paranoid woman rushed into another room when the social worker and doctor arrived. He felt powerless to deal with the situation and needed to be encouraged to take part in the interview. To exclude him could have served to emphasise his powerlessness whereas if he was included he could perhaps play a vital and enabling part in his wife's treatment and recovery.

There are many different models of crisis intervention services available. However, we should not forget that another definition of the word 'crisis' is 'turning-point'; it brings opportunities for change. The assessment interview might be seen not simply as a way of deciding whether or not someone needs to go into hospital, but also as the beginning of some real help for the client and family.

The presenting problem

The presenting problem is that which is perceived by the referrer. It will often be highly charged and will, in most instances, require further exploration and clarification to ensure that the full extent of the problem is understood before arranging the assessment interview.

Case example

A 20 year-old student has been sitting on her bed staring out of the window for days. She has not spoken or dressed herself and her flatmates are becoming extremely anxious because she is not eating and they fear that she might jump out of the window.

When the referrer is closely involved with the client – that is, a carer, family member or friend – he or she should be encouraged to participate in the assessment interview. If this action meets with a refusal the reasons for non-participation should be understood by the social worker and explained to the client at the start of the interview. It is helpful to tell the client at the beginning of the interview who everyone present is, and why they are there.

The most important task is then to invite the client to state the problem as he or she perceives it. This should be done using simple and direct language such as 'A lot of people are concerned about you/friends are worried about you. I'd like to hear from you what has been happening'. It is also important to ask the client whether he or she understands why the social worker and the doctor have come to see him or her.

Engaging with the user

Every picture tells a story, and everything that happens during the interview will help the approved social worker put together a picture of the client and assess the extent of the problem. The client's initial responses, the state of his or her surroundings and his or her ability to put into words what he or she thinks has been happening will form the basis of helping to resolve the problem.

The social worker must be sensitive to the attitudes of everyone in the assessment and their effects on the client. For example, when the husband rushed into another room in the case example on page 9, the social worker should notice the effect of this on the wife, draw attention to her husband's absence and either encourage her to help bring him back into the room or say why she prefers him to remain outside.

Of course, some clients will clearly be too disturbed to be able to engage with the social worker and doctor. In such cases, it will be necessary to understand what their 'normal' behaviour is like. The client may be in a florid, disturbed state and what he or she says may make no immediate sense whatsoever. The social worker should not pretend to understand the incomprehensible. He or she may be encountering a confused and confusing person with very bizarre beliefs and only experience will help develop the capacity to recognise and respond to the sane parts of a person's mind amid so much disorder.

At the other extreme, the client might make no response at all. Once again, the social worker needs to discover the significance of this and talk to someone who knows the client. It is important not to presume that an unresponsive and silent client is out of touch with what is going on, merely because he or she makes no verbal or visual contact. Even when someone is suffering from acute catatonic schizophrenia and appears to be completely mute and withdrawn he or she will be aware of what is going on and will be able to remember what has happened.

There is no doubt that one potentially difficult type of client to engage with is the paranoid person who may interpret any approach with suspicion. Such a client might well perceive those who have been called to them with suspicion and refuse to cooperate with the assessment. Alternatively, they may be relieved because their persecutory voices have given them a hard time, so may view the social worker and doctor as helping agents who will rescue him or her from his or her persecutors. This will usually be the case if he or she has had previously good contact with the hospital/social worker/

doctor or he or she can be reassured that the assessment is in his or her best interests.

Cultural factors

In a mixed society such as ours, the social worker needs to be aware of the additional stresses experienced by clients from ethnic minorities and the increased problems of communication, understanding of roles and attitudes to authority.

History

The client and his or her family should be asked to tell the social worker what he or she feels to be the important facts in the past associated with the present difficulties. He or she should also be asked about what and whom they found helpful. The doctor and the community psychiatric nurse will be able to provide medical history and give information about recent changes in medical and nursing management and the effects of any medication which the client may be taking. Non-compliance with medication invariably leads to a relapse and this can often be the primary reason for the client's present crisis. This is particularly important in the case of clients with a history of schizophrenia who are usually on regular medication. An understanding of why the client has stopped medication and his or her fears about continuing should be discussed with the client and his or her family and shared with the doctor and nurse. The CPA keyworker is the ideal person with whom to discuss the general status of the care plan and should be included in the assessment whenever possible.

Decision on action

The formulation of the decision on action will have to draw on the risk factors, the range of options and the client's motivation. When the social worker has been called on with the view to compulsory admission under the Mental Health Act the risk factor is central to the assessment process.

The approved social worker has to decide whether the client ought to be detained in hospital, either in the interests of his or her own health and safety or with a view to the protection of other persons (section 2 (2) (6)).

Someone with severe mental health problems who is destructive, either to themselves or others, is clearly recognisable as being in danger. However, the suicidal person is much less easy to recognise, and the degree of his or her depression will determine the level of risk. It is wise to use a direct approach, take time to talk to the client and ask whether he or she has considered ending his or her life. Such an open approach will usually facilitate an honest response in which the client will elaborate on how he or she will try to do this. This will help the social worker assess the seriousness of the risk of suicide.

The CPA keyworker, or other professionals and carers, should also be consulted for they are likely to be able to offer information about the current CPA status.

It may be more difficult to elicit the suicidal intent of a psychotic client for, as well as experiencing depression, he or she may be suffering delusions, as part of the psychotic process, which may contain the content of his or her suicidal thinking. For example the client may believe that his or her persecutors are coming to annihilate them and that the only way out is to commit suicide. Such frightening delusions can often be experienced by the client without anyone else being aware of them. These clients need skilled interviewing by experienced psychiatrists as part of the mental health assessment.

Of course, it may not be just suicide that occupies the psychotic client's thoughts, homicide may also feature as part of his or her delusional experience, and this will require careful and skilled intervention to assess the risk of murder and other potential acts of violence.

People with mental illness, like those who are physically ill, need effective and prompt help and treatment if they are not to deteriorate. The approved social worker must be aware of people who have become frightened and fragmented and feel alienated from all sources of safety. Such clients can go unnoticed or be regarded as social outcasts who do not require medical treatment but have 'chosen' this mode of living. Without appropriate help and treatment these clients can deteriorate further. Their 'welfare' may be much more at risk than the obviously violent or floridly ill person. Growing recognition of this issue has given rise to the development of 'assertive outreach teams' whose function is to sustain contact with service users who are outside the range of normal service provision.

The approved social worker has a responsibility to apply for admission if he or she is satisfied that the client is at risk and that hospitalisation is the most appropriate way of providing the care and medical treatment the client needs. A decision can only be made following an assessment of what is happening, what alternatives to hospital care are available to the client as a right and, most importantly, the likelihood of the client accepting whatever help is available.

Mental health: the law and practice

In this section we will set out the main provisions of the Mental Health Act 1983, the care programme approach, the Mental Health (Patients in the

Community) Act 1995, the concept of supervised discharge and supervision registers.

The Mental Health Act 1983

Admission for assessment in an emergency (section 4)

> **Case example**
>
> An approved social worker is called in by a police doctor at 3.00am to assess someone who has approached his or her neighbour for 'supplies'. The neighbour is worried and calls the police. In the assessment interview it emerges that the person is planning to drive to Egypt immediately without stopping. He has a car, but no licence and believes himself to be invulnerable – that is, he will not be stopping at traffic lights. The GP is not known and the district psychiatric hospital is some 20 miles away. In this example, the police doctor, in his or her capacity as a registered medical practitioner, could sign the medical recommendation for section 4. This then gives the ASW authority to make the application and request police assistance if necessary to escort the person to hospital.

Section 4 may be invoked on the same ground as section 2 (see below), the difference being that it is an urgent necessity that the patient be detained and that undertaking an assessment under section 2 would cause undesirable delay. Application can be made by an approved social worker or the nearest relative, and it is founded, if practicable, on a signed medical recommendation of one doctor who knows the patient – for example, his or her GP. Both the applicant and the doctor must have personally seen the patient during the 24 hours immediately prior to the application. Section 4 lasts for 72 hours, but within that time can be converted into sections either for admission for assessment (section 2), or treatment (section 3).

The use of section 4 by approved social workers is probably quite rare; unless the client is homeless, or not known, or the situation takes place outside the client's usual neighbourhood, access can normally be gained to his or her GP or an approved social worker. If these professionals are available it is always preferable to use sections 2 and 3, since they allow for more appropriate means of assessment and, if necessary, treatment for the distressed user.

Assessment (section 2)

If, in the case example above, a second medical opinion had been available or if the user was threatening to leave immediately and could be contained until the GP could be found, then section 2 would be the more appropriate section of the Act to consider.

Section 2 may be invoked where the patient is suffering from 'a mental disorder of a nature or degree which warrants his detention in hospital for assessment (or for the assessment followed by medical treatment) and he ought to be detained in the interests of his own health and safety or with a view to the protection of others'. Application may be made by an approved social worker or the nearest relative, founded on two medical recommendations, one of which must be made by a doctor approved by the Secretary of State 'as having special experience in the diagnosis and treatment of mental disorder' (section 12). The other medical recommendation should preferably be made by a doctor who knows the patient. If the doctors are making their examinations separately, no more than five days should elapse between each examination. Section 2 is normally used in situations where the patient is not known to the special psychiatric services or where it is judged that the patient's condition has changed since previous admission and he or she needs further assessment.

In making the application the approved social worker should take practicable steps to inform the nearest relative of the application, and of his or her right to order the patient's discharge. However, there is no obligation to obtain the nearest relative's agreement prior to making the application.

Application for hospital admission must be made within 14 days of the second medical recommendation. The patient may be detained for up to 28 days from the time of application.

Treatment (section 3)

Section 3 of the Mental Health Act can be invoked when it is necessary to detain someone in hospital under medical supervision; this can include 're-habilitation, habilitation and medical treatment'. It can be used where informal admission is inappropriate or in respect of someone already in hospital informally – for example under sections 2 or 4 or subject to guardianship.

An application for admission for treatment under section 3 (2) may be made on the following grounds:

1 the person is suffering from mental illness, severe mental impairment, psychopathic disorder or mental impairment and his or her mental disorder is of a nature or degree which makes it appropriate for him or her to receive medical treatment in hospital; and

2 in the case of psychopathic disorder or mental impairment, such treatment is likely to alleviate or prevent a deterioration of his or her condition; and

3 it is necessary for the health and safety of the patient or for the protection

of others that he or she receive such treatment and it cannot be provided unless he or she is detained under this section.

Admission for treatment (section 3)

Treatability requirement Admission under section 3 in respect of someone with a psychopathic disorder or mental impairment can only be made if the medical recommendation confirms that 'such treatment is likely to alleviate or prevent a deterioration of his condition' and is necessary for the health and safety or for the protection of other people.

Treatment need not be expected to cure the patient's disorder and a patient can be admitted under section 3 if, in the opinion of the doctors making the medical recommendations, medical treatment is likely to enable the patient to cope more satisfactorily with his or her disorder or its symptoms, or if it prevents his or her condition from deteriorating.

For example, a patient may need to be admitted to hospital for treatment due to a crisis necessitating medication or care, during a stressful life event or during a period of marked deterioration, even if treatment is unlikely to improve the actual mental impairment or mental illness. However, any renewal of the treatment order can only be made on certain criteria.

Medical recommendations Two medical recommendations are needed and the general provisions as to medical recommendations apply as follows:

- Only one of the medical recommendations may come from a practitioner or the staff of the hospital to which the patient is to be admitted or detained, except under very exceptional circumstances (see section 12 (4)).
- Where possible, the other medical recommendation should be made by a doctor with previous knowledge of the patient. In the case of private patients the medical recommendations may not be from doctors or the staff of the hospital.
- Both the medical recommendations must include a clinical description of the patient's mental condition, and each recommendation must describe the patient as having one of the same form of disorder, although any of the recommendations may list more than one disorder.
- The medical recommendations for admission under section 3 must also contain a statement as to whether alternatives to admission are available and, if so, why are they not used. They must also state the reasons why informal admission is not appropriate. The medical recommendations have to be completed before an application for admission is made, and the doctors making the recommendations must have

personally examined the patient, together or separately, not more than five days apart if the examinations are made separately.
- For the purpose of supplying a medical recommendation, a GP employed part-time in a hospital is not regarded as a member of the hospital staff (section 12 (6)).
- Where one recommendation is made by a consultant the other may not be made by a doctor who works for him or her.

Application   An application for admission under Section 3 can be made by:

1   **An approved social worker.** This can be an approved social worker acting outside the area in which he or she is appointed.
2   **The nearest relative.** The applicant must have seen the patient within 14 days ending with the date of the application, and the application has to be supported by two medical recommendations.

The social report   When the application for admission for treatment is made by the nearest relative, the hospital managers must inform the local social services authority for the area in which the patient resided in immediately before his or her admission. The social services authority must, as soon as practicable, arrange for a social worker to interview the patient and provide the managers with a report on his or her social circumstances (section 14).

The social worker making the social circumstances report does not have to be an approved social worker. The report should include the patient's social history, family accommodation, employment and finances as well as the suitability and availability of community resources.

Sometimes there may be doubt as to which social services authority should make the social circumstances report, particularly in respect of a patient of no fixed abode or admitted from temporary accommodation, such as a homeless person's hostel or squat. The Act refers to the 'area in which the patient resided immediately before his admission'. A patient's last 'residence' could therefore be his or her marital home or parent's address, provided that he or she intended to return there.

The relatives' right to be consulted   An approved social worker who makes an application under section 3 of the Mental Health Act is required to take reasonably practicable steps to consult the nearest relative, if there is one, either before, or within reasonable time after, the application, and advise the relative of the application and his or her right to object. Contact with the relative could be made either personally by the approved social worker, by telephone or letter, or by someone acting on behalf of the approved social worker – for example, a social worker in another district covering the relative's address.

The nearest relative does not have to consent to the admission but must, if practicable, be informed and be made aware of his or her right to object. The application for admission under section 3 cannot be made if the nearest relative signifies his objection (section 11 (4)).

Documents The applicant is responsible for the delivery of the admission documents to the managers of the hospital, and the application form, which should be delivered by hand, must arrive before or at the time of the admission.

The application form contains the following requirements:

1 If neither of the medical practitioners knew the patient before the medical recommendations were made, the applicant must state why it was not possible to obtain a recommendation from a medical practitioner who *did* know the patient prior to the date of the application.

2 If the application is made by an approved social worker he or she must state either:

   a) that he or she has consulted the nearest relative who has not notified any objection to the application; or

   b) it is not reasonably practicable to consult the nearest relative or the nearest relative is not known and there appears to be no relative; and

   c) that he or she has interviewed the patient and is satisfied that detention in a hospital is, in all the circumstances of the case, the most appropriate way of providing the care and medical treatment that the patient needs.

The patient must be admitted to hospital within 14 days of the second medical recommendation.

Duration An admission under section 3 is, in the first instance, for a period of six months.

Renewal The responsible medical officer has a duty, within two months of the end of detention period, to examine the patient and if he or she is satisfied that the patient should remain in hospital, must complete a Renewal of Authority for Detention (Form 30) addressed to the hospital managers.

Before making a report for Renewal of the Authority for Detention the responsible medical officer must consult one or more other persons who have been professionally concerned with the patient's treatment. The Act does not specify that these have to be professionals from other disciplines, and the decision as to whom to consult is that of the responsible medical officer (section

20 (5)). In order to renew a treatment order under section 3 all of the following must apply:

1   The patient is suffering from mental illness, severe mental impairment, psychopathic disorder or mental impairment and his or her mental disorder is of a nature or degree that makes it appropriate for him or her to receive medical treatment in hospital.
2   Such treatment is likely to alleviate or prevent a deterioration of his or her condition.
3   It is necessary for the health and safety of the patient or for the protection of others that he or she should receive treatment and that it cannot be provided unless he or she continues to be detained.

In the case of mental illness or severe mental impairment, a treatment order under section 3 may be renewed if, in the opinion of the responsible medical officer, the patient would be unlikely to care for himself or herself, to obtain the care that he or she needs or guard against serious exploitation (section 20 (4)). This section prevents patients who are unlikely to be able to care for themselves from being discharged from hospital unless there are suitable alternatives. A patient cannot be detained under section 3 if he or she is willing and able to remain in hospital as an informal patient. The hospital managers must inform the nearest relative, if there is one, and the patient, that the order has been renewed.

Medical treatment   A patient admitted to hospital under section 3 can be given certain types of treatment without consent. This is governed by the Code of Practice issued by the Secretary of State and covered by sections 56 and 64. A patient can be given a course of medication or drug treatment without his or her consent for a period up to three months, after which the psychiatrist in charge of his treatment has to make an evaluation of the treatment and consider the long-term treatment programme. In the case of an emergency, a patient can, like any non-psychiatric patient, be given treatment for a medical condition without his or her consent if such treatment is essential.

Mental health review tribunals   The patient has a right to apply to a mental health review tribunal at any time within the first six months of his or her detention in hospital. If he or she withdraws the application, he or she can apply again. If the order is renewed, the patient can apply once again in the second six months and once in every subsequent 12 months (section 66). If the patient does not personally apply to the tribunal after six months, the hospital managers must apply to the tribunal on his behalf.

Discharge   A treatment order under section 3 is discharged in the following circumstances.

1   **At the natural expiration of the period of the order if not renewed.** That is, at the end of the first six months, at the end of the second six months, at the end of each subsequent year.
2   **By order of the nearest relative.** The nearest relative must give 72 hours' notice in writing, or by form 34, addressed to the hospital managers, of his or her intention to discharge the patient (section 25 (1)).

   The nearest relative can arrange for a doctor to see the patient and examine him or her in private for the purpose of advising as to discharge. The responsible medical officer if he or she considers that, in his or her opinion, the patient, if discharged, would be likely to act in a manner dangerous to him or herself or others, can issue a report barring discharge to the nearest relative (Form 36). In this case, the nearest relative must be informed and cannot order discharge for a further six months although he or she has the right to apply to the review tribunal to consider discharge.
3   **By order of the responsible medical officer or by the hospital managers.**
4   **By order of the Secretary of State.** This applies if the patient is detained in a mental nursing home or, if the patient is maintained under contract with the health authority, by that authority.
5   **By decision of the mental health review tribunal.** The patient has the right to apply to the tribunal at any time within the first six months, once during the next six months and yearly thereafter. He or she can be legally represented. He or she can ask the tribunal to consider his or her case by writing to them or the hospital managers.
6   **If reclassified by the responsible medical officer.** If the patient is reclassified as suffering from a mental disorder other than that specified in the application the authority to detain the patient ceases. Should the responsible medical officer reclassify the patient as suffering from a major to minor disorder, from a previous major disorder, he or she must state whether the treatability requirement is fulfilled. If it is not, the authority for detention will cease.
7   **If the patient is absent from the hospital without authority or trace for 28 days.**
8   After a continuous period of six months' leave of absence from the hospital.

Leave of absence from hospital (section 17)   The responsible medical officer can allow the patient to leave the hospital subject to whatever conditions he or she considers necessary in the interests of the patient or other people. He or she may either grant an indefinite period of leave or specify its exact duration.

A planned period of leave from the hospital can be a valuable means of rehabilitating a patient being considered for discharge. The responsible medical officer can recall a patient at any time by giving notice in writing to the patient or carer. He or she can also offer support to the carer during the trial period. A patient on continuous leave for a period of six months is no longer liable to be detained in hospital.

Other compulsory powers

Of particular relevance to social workers are three other provisions contained in the Mental Health Act 1983 concerning statutory powers. These are:

- section 5 (2), doctor's holding power
- section 5 (4), nurse's holding power
- section 115, concerned with approved social workers' right of entry
- section 135, which is a warrant to enter and remove a patient from his or her home
- section 136, which relates to mentally disordered persons found in public places.

These powers are examined in more detail below.

Section 5 (2)   Under this section, an informal patient in a psychiatric hospital or a general hospital may be detained for up to 72 hours if the doctor in charge of the treatment reports that an application for 'admission' ought to be made. The 72 hours takes effect from the time the report is received by the hospital managers. A second medical recommendation must be obtained during this time period, so that an approved social worker can proceed with assessment and, if appropriate, application for section 2 or 3. If the patient leaves hospital he or she may be retaken within 72 hours of the doctor's report.

Section 5 (4)   Under this part of the section, a first-level nurse (a registered mental health nurse) may detain an informal patient who is already being treated for mental disorder for a period not more than six hours, if it appears to him or her that:

1   the patient is suffering from mental disorder to such a degree that it is necessary for the health and safety or protection of others for him or her to be immediately restrained from leaving the hospital;
2   it is not practicable to secure the immediate attendance of a medical practitioner for the purpose of furnishing a report under section 5 (2).

The 'holding' power starts after the nurse has recorded his or her opinion on the prescribed form (Form 13) and this ends six hours later, or on the earlier arrival of one of the two doctors (that is, the responsible medical officer in charge of the case or nominated deputy) entitled to make a report under section 5 (2). The doctor is free to make such a report or to decide not to detain the patient further (which may, for example, include persuading him or her to stay voluntarily). The six hours' holding period counts as part of the 72 hours, if the doctor concerned decides to make a report under section 5 (2). If the patient leaves hospital he or she may be retaken within six hours of the nurse's recorded opinion.

Section 115   Section 115 empowers an approved social worker of a local authority social services to enter and inspect any premises (not a hospital) in the area of that authority in which a mentally disordered person is living, if the social worker has reasonable cause to believe that the patient is not under proper care.

This power applies 'at all reasonable times', which will depend on the urgency of the situation. It is not a power to use force of entry. If entry is refused, caution may be given that such refusal constitutes an offence under section 129 of the Act (which states that any person who forbids an inspection of premises, or an assessment under the Act, or other obstruction without reasonable cause, commits an offence). If, after the due caution, entry is still refused, the approved social worker may apply for a warrant of entry, under section 135 of the Act.

Section 135   An approved social worker may obtain, from the Justice of the Peace, a warrant enabling a constable to enter the premises and search for and remove a patient if there is 'reasonable cause to suspect that a person believed to be suffering from mental disorder' has been ill-treated, neglected, has not been kept under proper control, or is unable to care for himself or herself and living alone. The warrant must name the constable who is to enter the premises, and the constable must be accompanied by both an approved social worker and a registered medical practitioner.

Section 136   A police officer may remove to a place of safety a person who appears to be suffering from mental disorder and is in immediate need of care and control and is in a place to which the public has access (for example, a theatre or public highway and so on). The person can be detained for 72 hours, so that he or she can be examined and assessed by a doctor and an approved social worker. The place of safety can be a police station or a hospital. It is important to note that the purpose of detention is not to provide custody, but to enable an assessment to be made. Once the assessment has been made, the authority for detention expires, even if 72 hours have not elapsed.

The care programme approach (CPA)

Under the NHS and Community Care Act 1990 there is a requirement for all patients under the care of the specialist mental health services to have a CPA; this includes users who have been treated in hospital and those who have been released from prison. Social services departments, together with the health authority and voluntary agencies, also have a legal responsibility under section 117 of the Mental Health Act 1983 to provide aftercare of users who have been subject to sections 3, 37, 47 and 48 of the Mental Health Act 1983.

The care programme approach extends the statutory duty of the health and social services and, if properly implemented, will fulfil the duties of the NHS and Community Care Act 1990, the legal requirements of section 117 Mental Health Act 1983, those users on the supervision register and those subject to supervised discharge under the Mental Health Act 1995.

The CPA has four main elements:

1   systematic assessment of the immediate and long-term health and social care needs of all patients who have been accepted by the specialist mental health services;
2   formulation of a care plan which has been agreed between relevant professionals, the patient and the carer;
3   the nomination of a named keyworker to keep in close contact and monitor the agreed care plan, ensuring that service delivery is coordinated;
4   the arrangement of appropriate reviews when necessary.

Specialist psychiatric services consist of a multidisciplinary team of professionals with particular skills in working with users with severe and enduring mental health problems. We have already stressed elsewhere the need to be able to work effectively together to share the burden of care. Often, because of the nature of mental illness, the user can confuse and split those involved in their care. Without a clear understanding of this process, workers can unwittingly mirror this behaviour, leading to further confusion and difficulty in communication. Sharing each other's perception and understanding of the user can sometimes minimise some of these issues. Most health and social services authorities have taken a layered or tiered approach to CPA, which takes into account the complexity of service users' needs and the degree of risk which they may pose to themselves or others. Users are assessed and assigned to one of the three levels of the CPA.

- **CPA level 1.** These users will be accepted by the specialist mental health services and will not normally need the care of the other two levels.
- **CPA level 2.** These will be users who have been accepted by the specialist mental health team and who require the care and support of multidisciplinary services. One or more of the following risk factors will apply.
  - The user has a severe mental illness which produces disabilities including those which make it very difficult to find suitable housing.
  - There is a history of repeated relapse due to the resumption of the user's illness and to the breakdown of medical and social care in the community.
- **CPA level 3.** These are users who meet one or more of the following criteria and who may be placed on the supervision register.
  - risk of severe self-harm and suicide attempts
  - risk of severe self-neglect
  - risk of danger to others
  - subject to supervised discharge.

The CPA keyworker

In the past the keyworker concept has been used in several settings – for example, in residential care settings to coordinate the work of residential staff. Keyworking has been more widely and successfully used in child protection work.

The keyworker's role within the context of the CPA has several important functions, including direct user care, user and carer involvement, interprofessional and interagency collaboration.

In summary, the keyworker's role is to ensure cooperation between professionals and agencies, maintain contact with the user and carer, make sure that the care plan is delivered satisfactorily and convene reviews of the care plan when necessary.

The choice of the keyworker will depend on a number of considerations, including staff availability and workload and the gender and ethnicity of the worker; clearly the user is more likely to comply with the care plan if the keyworker is someone he or she knows and trusts.

The Mental Health (Patients in the Community) Act 1995

The Mental Health (Patients in the Community) Act 1995 came into operation on 1 April 1996. It introduces the new provision of 'supervised discharge' and amends the Mental Health Act 1983. The main focus of the Act is the severely mentally ill who often show a pattern of relapse following discharge and, for this reason, are often referred to as the 'revolving door syndrome'. The aim of this legislation is to ensure that these patients receive the care services which should be provided under section 117 of the Mental Health Act 1983.

Criteria

1 Supervised discharge may only be applied to hospital inpatients who fulfil the following criteria:
   - The patient must be over 16 *and*
   - is currently detained under sections 3, 37, 47 of the Mental Health Act 1983.

2 The patient must be suffering from one or more of the four broad categories of mental disorder identified in section 1 (2) of the Mental Health Act 1983, namely:
   - mental illness
   - mental impairment
   - severe mental impairment
   - psychopathic disorder.

3 There are two tests which will require the judgement of the professionals concerned:
   - There would be substantial risk of serious harm to the health or safety of the patient or of other people, or the patient being seriously exploited if the patient did not receive aftercare services under section 117 of the Mental Health Act 1983.
   - Supervision is likely to help ensure that the patient received these services.

Procedure

The supervision application is made by the resident medical officer (RMO) who is usually the consultant psychiatrist in charge of the patient's care (or someone they expressly nominate). He or she must consult with the following people before making an application in order to give them a genuine opportunity to offer comment on the proposed arrangements and to take their views into account:

- the patient
- the hospital team
- the community team

- voluntary agencies
- the informal carer
- the nearest relative.

The 'key point of difference' is that the RMO is the applicant, in contrast to other sections of the Mental Health Act 1983 where the applicant is usually the approved social worker. However, the RMO's application must be accompanied by written recommendations by an approved social worker and the doctor who will be professionally involved in the patient's care in the community. This will give the approved social worker the opportunity and scope to inspect the patient's medical records and interview the patient before deciding to make a recommendation as well as to look at the patient's rights and the wider social issues. All three parties must agree before the application can proceed.

Powers

The requirements placed on patients will be included in the care plan. A patient may be required:

- to reside at a specific place
- to attend a particular place at set times for medical treatment, occupation or training
- to allow access to their home to the supervisor, any registered medical practitioner or any approved social worker or any other person authorised by the supervisor.

The supervisor, or any person authorised by the supervisor, may convey the patient to their designated home but there is no power to detain him or her. Likewise, the patient can be conveyed for medical treatment but cannot be treated without his or her consent.

The role of the supervisor   The supervisor must be an experienced and qualified member of the care team. His or her main responsibility is monitoring the progress of the care plan and ensuring that patients comply with the requirements placed on them by the Act – that is, residence, attendance and convening reviews with other members of the care team when they are due.

How can the supervision end?   Supervision may end under the following circumstances:

- after the RMO has consulted the supervisor and patient and directed that the patient ceases to be subject to supervision

- if the patient is readmitted to hospital under section 3 or received into guardianships
- when the patient is remanded or committed into custody, for as long as he or she is detained
- if the patient is absent without leave for a period longer than six months
- if the mental health review tribunal discharges the order.

Duration

Supervised discharge is for an initial period of six months and is renewable for a further period of six months and annually thereafter.

The supervision register

The supervision register was introduced in April 1994 for those patients subject to CPA who are at most risk to themselves or others. It aims to ensure that patients receive sufficiently adequate care, support and supervision in the community to prevent them from falling through the care network.

Categories of inclusion

At the time of inclusion, and at each subsequent review at which the patient is left on the register, patients will be assigned to one or more of the following categories:

- significant risk of suicide
- significant risk of violence to others
- significant risk of severe neglect.

Where the risk of committing serious violence, suicide or severe self-neglect is considered to be linked to specific events, such as stopping medication, the loss of a supportive relationship or the loss of accommodation, the identified warning signs should be recorded.

When is the risk assessment completed?

The risk assessment is completed:

- at the initial assessment
- at the CPA meeting
- at subsequent CPA reviews
- during all hospital admissions.

Who decides if someone is placed on the register?

The decision as to who is placed on the register rests with the consultant psychiatrist responsible for the patient's care. This decision should be made in consultation with other members of the mental health team (which includes the social worker involved in the care).

What will the patient be told?

The patient will be told:

- why he or she has been placed on the register
- how the information will be used
- to whom the information may be disclosed
- of the right of appeal.

Right of appeal The patient and his or her advocate will have the right to request verbally or in writing removal from the register. The consultant psychiatrist, in conjunction with professional colleagues, will consider these requests and inform the patient of the outcome and reasons for the decision. If a patient remains dissatisfied, he or she has the right of a second opinion and, if this course is taken, all assistance will be given.

Who can request removal from the register?

Any of the agencies or professionals involved in the care plan may request a special meeting to consider removal. The patient will be given the opportunity to attend the meeting, and if he or she wishes, an advocate, relative, friend or carer can accompany him or her to state his or her views and have them fully considered.

When will the patient be taken off the register?

The patient's continued inclusion on the register should be considered at every review. A copy of the register entry will be sent to the keyworker before the CPA review and alterations can be made on that.

Patients will be taken off the register if they are no longer assessed as being a risk to themselves or others. This decision can only be made at the review meeting.

Who has access to the register?

The patient has a legal right to access his or her own records, subject to essential safeguards under the Access to Health Records Act 1990 and Data Protection Act 1984. In addition, mental health professionals have access on a need-to-know basis, as does the patient's GP who will inform members of the primary health team, again on a need-to-know basis.

Disclosure to other agencies, social services departments, the probation service, police and so on may be made with the patient's agreement or without, if disclosure can be justified to be in the public interest.

Visiting members of the Mental Health Act Commission have access to records on detained persons.

A record is kept of all who have had access to the data and when.

Notes on structure

Over recent years, social work and health services have become increasingly decentralised. The old jigsaw comprised the remote asylum, designed for long-stay patients and fed from a combination of satellite villages and inner cities. Although, sometimes, asylums had acute facilities, acute beds would often be based in the local general hospital, known as the district general hospital. Social workers (originally known as almoners) would be based in the asylum as well as in local fieldwork teams, known as area offices. In area offices, social workers would be referred to as 'generic social workers'. This term reflected the generalist nature of their work, generalism being a founding tenet of the Seebohm reforms which moved social work away from specialism towards the general practitioner model. The Seebohm Report was published in 1968 and enacted in the reorganisation of social services in 1970.

The Mental Health Act 1983 reintroduced some concept of specialism with the introduction of the approved social worker although, at inception, this role was adopted by many generic field social workers. The period since 1983 has seen a profound shift in attitudes, policy and law, simultaneously – and paradoxically – away from ideas of genericism and towards specialisation, yet also towards decentralisation and towards interdisciplinary teamwork and collaboration.

Certainly in relation to mental health services, most local social services and health authorities now provide locality teams, combining professionals from several diverse disciplines – predominantly social work and community psychiatric nursing, with sessional input usually from a consultant psychiatrist, possibly a psychologist and possibly an occupational therapist. Instead of feeding patients through a system involving remote asylums, such teams have now developed the practice of integrating hospital admissions on a sector basis and remaining involved with service users as they pass through the psychiatric system through from admission, treatment to aftercare.

Theoretically, this should provide continuity of care and a safety net to guarantee care on discharge for the service user; this is the way in which authorities attempt to discharge their responsibilities to provide aftercare, care programming and supervised discharge. The system relies, however, on a number of factors which are sometimes not there. Chief amongst such factors are:

1 good interprofessional collaboration, rather than infighting and competitiveness (hence the discussions and examples referred to earlier in this chapter)
2 sufficient hospital beds to avoid having to transport service users vast distances out of the district when no local beds are available and extra-contractual referrals have to be agreed
3 sufficient hospital beds to enable beds to be available when necessary or, when this is not possible, ready access to decisions about extracontractual referrals to prevent unwarrantable delay that places workers and clients (and relatives and/or the public) at risk
4 clear lines of accountability and responsibility to allow workers to feel that they are supported if they take risks
5 sufficient alternatives to admission should someone need a place of safety that is not necessarily a hospital
6 culturally sensitive services – in the hospital and community – so that service users, and relatives, feel that their individual issues and circumstances can be recognised and valued.

2 Psychiatry, diagnosis and treatment

Introduction

Psychiatric disorders are the third most common reason for consultation in general practice. Over 90 per cent of mentally ill people are seen by their GP but are not always treated or referred to specialist psychiatric services. Yet one of the most crucial factors in mental health is the need to make an early diagnosis so that treatment can be introduced as soon as possible in order to prevent further deterioration.

In this chapter we will be looking at the wide range of mental disorders from the milder neuroses to the major psychotic disorders which will often become the main concern of the approved social worker. In addition, we have included a description of the physical and psychological treatments which are now available.

Within the hospital setting the multidisciplinary team is responsible for planning the care and treatment of the patient. The core team is led by the consultant psychiatrist (the RMO), his or her senior registrar and senior house officer, who are usually responsible for the daily medical care and supervision of patients, a ward nurse, a community psychiatric nurse (CPN), an occupational therapist, a psychologist and a social worker. The members of the team keep in close liaison, the core members meeting together weekly in ward rounds and other meetings, to monitor the patient's care and progress.

Ultimate responsibility for the patient's care lies with the consultant psychiatrist who, in the terms of the Mental Health Act 1983, is designated the responsible medical officer (RMO). The tasks of each member of the multidisciplinary team complement one another so as to provide a coherent care plan. In the past, the social worker was seen as the 'bridge' between the hospital and the community. With the CPA the hospital and community are seen as a seamless service, so this role is shared with other professionals. In practice it is often the patient's needs which decide which professional is nominated as the keyworker. For example, if the patient has difficulty in complying with medication, a CPN may be seen as the most appropriate member to act as keyworker, whereas, if the patient's needs are predominately social, the social worker will be nominated. Obviously, the process is often more subtle than this, and issues of gender, culture and skills may need to be considered when deciding who should become the nominated keyworker. The CPA meeting should include the patient's carer, who can be by far the greatest resource in supporting the patient. In addition, local voluntary agencies involved in mental health should be included. The care programme approach has been dealt with in more detail in Chapter 1.

Psychiatric illness

Most of us, from time to time, experience emotional distress and, indeed, may regard this as normal. The degree of emotional suffering that many of our clients suffer can sometimes be related to external causes in their lives.

Here, we begin by looking at the major patterns of distress as they are classified in terms of psychiatric illness. We will first consider the milder forms of mental disorder, the psychoneuroses, in which the sufferer can experience considerable and lasting difficulties which severely impair his or her ability to cope. We will then go on to consider the psychotic disorders in which the personality is profoundly disturbed.

Neuroses

The neuroses are the milder psychiatric disorders. Reality is less distorted than is the case with psychoses, and insight is retained. The four main groups are:

- anxiety states
- obsessional compulsive disorders
- hysteria
- reactive or neurotic depression.

Anxiety states

Anxiety is a normal enough state for most of us to understand. Indeed, the anxiety states are probably the most common of all psychiatric disorders and make up a large proportion of complaints which bring patients to consult their GPs. Someone suffering from an anxiety neurosis is likely to complain of a number of symptoms, ranging from mild apprehension to feelings of acute panic. Many describe an almost constant state of anxiety, where there are physical sensations of choking and fears of going out alone or into crowded places such as restaurants. Such fears can sometimes make it impossible for a person to function. A feeling of 'free-floating' anxiety may be felt for no apparent reason.

In other cases, physical symptoms of headaches, palpitations and frequency of urination may be present. If patients believe that they have a diseased organ, for which there is no medical evidence, this is called hypochondriasis. Behind many complaints of headache and lack of sleep brought to GPs, there is an underlying anxiety state. It should, however, be stressed that worry is normal. It motivates us to take action and make decisions, but worry that overwhelms and is undefined can inhibit and seriously impair the sufferer.

Treatment

Clinically, most neurotic anxiety is seen and dealt with by the GP rather than the psychiatrist. Treatment can take the form of reassurance and support for minor complaints, progressing to outpatient psychotherapy or counselling.

These processes can enable patients to gain understanding and insight into the underlying conflicts which may be sustaining these symptoms.

Obsessional compulsive disorders

Most of us will be familiar with the experience of having a tune that goes around and around in our head, or a senseless idea which occurs repeatedly. With the obsessive patient such experiences are felt to a crippling degree. These obsessions often take the form of thoughts which are intrusive and keep occurring in the patient's mind against his or her will. These thoughts can often be of a violent or obscene nature or contain fears of contamination.

Compulsions take root as a response to these thoughts. They are irresistible urges to perform an act or a protective ritual in an attempt to ward off the anxiety that such thoughts generate. Obsessive patients fear that, if they do not carry out these rituals, they will face retribution such as eternal damnation. The most common compulsive acts are checking and handwashing. Sufferers can become preoccupied for hours, checking and rechecking to see whether they have turned off gas taps. This can extend to checking doors and windows until most of the day is taken up with such activity. Handwashing is a ritual which is often related to contamination. The patient usually has a special way of washing, and this can be repeated up to 40 times a day until the intense anxiety diminishes. Furthermore, the number of times the patient needs to perform the ritual can often take on a magical significance.

The type of person most prone to this disorder is likely to have been described as 'a very worthy citizen' as he or she is neat, tidy and orderly. However, such individuals tend to be too rigid and carry their desire for orderliness too far. Their behaviour can put considerable strain on friends and relatives. To try to prevent patients from carrying out rituals can only increase their anxiety, which leads in turn to an increase in the compulsive behaviour. People who seem to be most vulnerable to developing such disorders are those who have obsessive personalities.

Treatment

Treatment may be in the form of medication; tranquillisers may be prescribed to ease some of the more distressing symptoms associated with these disorders. They do little, however, to alter the underlying causes.

Psychosurgery is sometimes prescribed for patients who have suffered this illness for a long time and for those with such severe symptoms that they cripple their ability to live life in any meaningful or satisfactory way.

In less severe cases, behaviour therapy might be considered. In cases where there is an obsessional compulsive component, which is diffused and generalised rather than converted into a specific symptom, psychotherapy may be considered. An example would be a patient with the feeling that everything must be checked two or three times, but then considers that it is safe, as contrasted with a patient who cannot actually move away from a door for several hours because he or she is not sure, but must check repeatedly, that it is locked.

Hysteria

Hysteria, as a term, is now in general parlance to describe someone who is 'out of control', or it is sometimes used incorrectly as a term of abuse. The word derives from the Latin *hystericus* which means 'of the womb'. Many of the symptoms of hysteria are found more commonly in women; these are unconsciously motivated and can often mimic physical illness. It is therefore crucial that a thorough medical examination is carried out to eliminate any physical basis for the symptoms.

Conversion hysteria

A hysterical conversion symptom usually involves the sensory or motor systems of the body. It has no neurological basis but is in response to some unconscious psychological conflict and often provides some 'gain' for the sufferer. Such gains can be divided into:

- **Primary gain.** First described by Freud, this gives relief from some intolerable intrapsychic conflict.
- **Secondary gain.** This involves demanding help or allowing the patient to escape from some stressful situation. Such hysterical symptoms are manifold; they can, for example, include paralysis, tremor, deafness, blindness and fits.

Hysterical dissociation

This process is similar to hysterical conversion – that is, conflict followed by symptom formation. However, while the conversion symptoms involve the sensory/motor systems, hysterical dissociation involves narrowing the field of consciousness with selective amnesia (loss of memory).

Fugue (wandering states)

In this state, the patient may temporarily lead a double existence, adopting an alternative identity (a more extreme example being Dr Jekyll and Mr Hyde). Alternatively, the patient may suddenly find himself or herself in London, away from his or her familiar home in Newcastle, with no memory of why or how he or she arrived there. In other words, the process is unconscious and can be seen as a flight from a painful and stressful situation which the individual wants to escape. Such patients often recall the events after a period of a few weeks with the aid of abreactive procedures.

Munchausen's syndrome

This is a dissociative state in which the patient simulates signs of organic disease; or, in the case of Munchausen's by Proxy, stimulates illness or injury in children or adults in their care. Such individuals are sufficiently plausible as to engender extensive investigation, surgery, or employment in the care sector. A Munchausen's by Proxy diagnosis may only come to light after unexplained injuries or even death, occur.

Hysteria and malingering

It is important to try to distinguish between hysteria and malingering. The hysterical conversion symptoms and dissociation have an unconscious conflict as an underlying cause, whereas the malingerer is consciously aware of his abnormal behaviour.

Treatment

The treatment of hysteria has two main approaches. Where the disability has been caused by traumatic experiences in the person's life, abreaction may be indicated. In this approach, the patient is given drugs or hypnosis to help him or her recall and relive the trauma. Dramatic improvements can sometimes occur when the patient re-experiences what are often painful events. In more entrenched conditions, where the hysterical symptoms are part of a more disturbed personality structure, more long-term help may be required in the form of psychotherapy which enables the patient to gain insight into the unconscious factors that are creating his or her difficulties. The patient and therapist can then work through towards a better adjustment.

Behaviour therapy is also a useful approach. Here the focus is on how the patient's secondary gain is helping sustain his illness – that is, what ends are being satisfied by being ill.

Reactive or neurotic depression

Neurotic depression is usually felt in response to a distressing experience of some kind. There is often some preoccupation with a psychic trauma which precedes the illness. Examples of this could be bereavement, the loss of a friend or relative or life changes such as retirement. Anxiety is also frequently present, and mixed states of anxiety and depression are included in the psychiatric definition.

It is important to distinguish between neurotic depression and psychotic depression. This is done on the basis of degree of depression, and also on the presence or absence of other neurotic and psychotic characteristics – for example, delusions and nihilistic beliefs – and on the degree of disturbance of the patient's behaviour.

The clinical classification of neurotic depression should not be confused with general or specific feelings of unhappiness which most people experience. This unhappiness can arise for many reasons and take many forms. Neurotic depression is a specific clinical description of a mental state.

What is depression?

Depression is a complex emotional state involving an interplay of feelings, such as fear and anger, which seem to turn themselves against each other producing a painful depressed mood. In addition, the person often experiences a slowing down of mental and physical processes. This is often accompanied by an overriding feeling of helplessness and an inability to change the situation. In more extreme cases the depressed person may believe that he or she deserves to be punished because he or she is wicked.

Because of the nature of the disorder the patient may feel unworthy and, because of this, fail to seek help but continue to suffer in silence. Alternatively, the depressed person may present more subtle symptoms such as aches and pains, and the underlying depression may remain unrecognised even by the skilled professional.

Depression is clearly not a simple condition but involves many factors – for instance, the individual's basic capacity to bear and cope with feelings of loss, intrapsychic conflict and external stresses. In the more severe conditions biochemical factors may also play a part.

Treatment

Medication can alleviate some of the worst feelings of a neurotic depression and can act as a holding mechanism until other therapeutic forces can take effect. Counselling and psychotherapy are two key treatments of neurotic depression.

Social work with the depressed patient

Depression has become an umbrella term to describe those painful emotional states associated with loss, stressful circumstances such as illness and unemployment, handicap and disturbed relationships. With some clients the cause of depression may not be so clear – for example, many patients experience depression as an almost permanent feature of their personality and it is increased in times of stress, while, with others, depression seems to appear from out of the blue and has no apparent external cause. Depression is a very variable condition and can range from feelings of profound sadness to severe states where the patient is stuporised, mute and inaccessible. Trigger factors such as loss and disappointment can precipitate depressive reactions and, even in the most severe states, painful life events can be traced to three months prior to the onset of the episode.

Most cases of this kind of depression are treated by GPs or psychiatrists on an outpatient arrangement, with a combination of anti-depressant medication and supportive psychotherapy. In the more severe cases electroconvulsive therapy (ECT) may be indicated.

The counselling relationship

Clearly, the external causes for the patient's depression need to be addressed. However, we must go further. The patient invariably feels bad about him or herself. Furthermore, he or she feels that others cannot tolerate them either, and this deep attitude often militates against understanding and help.

It is through the counselling relationship that the patient can begin to feel accepted and helped with what he or she feels is unbearable within him or herself. Through this the patient will gradually begin to experience the counsellor as someone who can accept and bear the patient's depression. The counsellor must bear some of the patient's psychic pain, in order to enable the patient to do so. This is the essential key to achieving this kind of change, for it is not until the patient is convinced that the feelings of 'badness' can be borne that he or she can begin to integrate them into his or her whole personality without being overwhelmed.

The counsellor may well meet a deep self-defeating attitude within the patient which can easily be turned against the counsellor or those who try to help him or her. The counsellor will need to help the patient work with this aspect of his or her personality if change is to take place. Through this process of working through these feelings, the patient will begin to realise that his or her negative side is not all-powerful and will see his or her anger, resentment and other deep negative parts for what they are – aspects of him or herself – and begin to integrate them alongside his or her more positive feelings.

Psychoses

The psychoses are the most severe forms of mental disorders. These conditions include schizophrenia, manic depression and the organic psychoses.

The personalities of individuals suffering from such disorders are often fundamentally disturbed and can often lead to very disorganised and disruptive behaviour. In the case of schizophrenia, for example, patients may hear voices (auditory hallucinations) and believe themselves to be the subject of some fantastic scheme (delusion).

These symptoms often create a nightmare world for the sufferers in which distortions of reality become so marked that they are unable to distinguish between what is real in their inner and outer world and what is delusional. Because the psychotic process confuses and distorts, it will lead to great confusion and bewilderment in such patients and all those around him or her. Such patients do not usually have insight whilst in the grip of their illness. However, with others, partial insight may be present.

Broadly speaking, the psychoses can be divided into those known as functional psychoses, which are normally of unknown aetiology, and organic psychoses in which there is evidence of transient or permanent brain damage.

The functional psychoses are subdivided into the affective disorders, in which the primary disturbance is of mood or affect, and schizophrenia in which disorders of thinking, emotion and behaviour occur. This schema is illustrated in Figure 2.1. We will look at organic psychoses in more detail in Chapter 6.

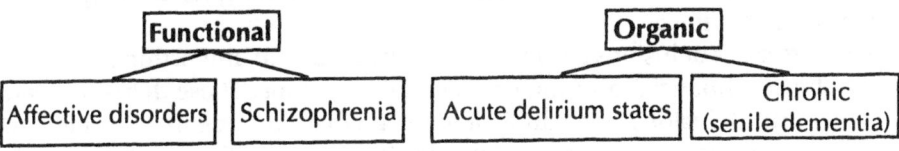

Figure 2.1   Psychoses

Functional psychoses: affective disorders

The main affective disorders are depression and mania. They can occur alone (unipolar) or they can alternate, forming the manic depressive cycle (bipolar). The bipolar disorder is usually recurring, often with long periods of remission during which the patient lives a normal life.

The most common disorder of mood is depression. It is the most severe type of depression and is called endogenous (psychotic) depression. The term means 'arising from within the person'. However, such depression can also be triggered off by life events which can sometimes be traced to events in the patient's life three months before the onset of the episode.

We will now trace the development of the depressive illness.

Psychotic depression

Here, the patient is profoundly depressed. If untreated the illness follows a characteristic course in which the depression and other presenting symptoms progress over a period of weeks until the maximum severity of the illness is reached. It may then remain for some time until a gradual improvement occurs.

Treatment in the form of antidepressant medication or ECT dramatically shortens each episode. In about 50 per cent of cases, there is no further episode but, in the remainder, there may be recurrences, and these may arise at critical times – for example, at childbirth or during other critical life events.

Depressed patients usually feel at their worst first thing in the morning when, characteristically, they awaken early; it is not until later in the day that they begin to feel slightly better. Their appetite is usually affected; they eat little and soon begin to lose weight. Their physical and mental activity is slowed down by a process known as retardation which is reflected in a marked slowness of thoughts, speech and body movements. On a mental level such patients will find it difficult to concentrate, think and make decisions. A marked loss of drive is present. They may withdraw from social contacts and their usual interests. They may become mute and inaccessible. There may also be increased anxiety which may manifest itself in agitation or restless behaviour.

In severe cases delusions occur. These can be related to unworthiness, moral worth, health, financial position or social relationships. These delusions can develop into delusions of a nihilistic nature wherein patients may believe that they are dead or that their insides are rotting away with cancer. Although patients may be quite wealthy, they may believe themselves to be poor or bankrupt. By far the most common delusions are those related to health and hypochrondias.

Suicide must always be regarded as a high risk. Patients may believe that life is not worth living and kill themselves. In very rare and extreme cases, they may murder their wives and children and then kill themselves.

Treatment

Because of the great risk of suicide such patients will need to be admitted to hospital – if necessary, on a compulsory order. Many psychiatrists see ECT as the first treatment of choice for such disorders, since antidepressant medication takes a few weeks before it becomes effective. Certainly the evidence suggests that this is the one condition which improves dramatically after ECT and, because of the urgent need to intervene, it will often be used first, perhaps alongside a course of antidepressant medication. Most psychiatrists now use lithium carbonate after the severe depression has lifted, both as an immediate remedy and as a more long-term preventive measure.

Mania or hypomania

Mania or hypomania is more commonly seen as a bipolar affective disorder – that is, as the manic phase of the manic depressive cycle in which manic states alternate with severe depressive episodes. Between these states there are often long periods of remission in which the patient is well and leads a normal life. Hypomania is much less common than depression.

In contrast to the depressive phase, manic patients are elated, carefree and apparently unconcerned. The degree of the disorder is variable – for example, they may initially just seem to be in a bouncy optimistic mood and the illness may progress considerably before relatives realise there is something wrong. Their moods may become euphoric and expansive, and an infectious sense of gaiety takes over.

There is considerable pressure of speech and flight of ideas so that patients swiftly pass from one topic to the next. They may then begin to express extraordinary ideas of their power and importance and these can soon develop into grandiose delusions. It is not uncommon for such patients to become involved in senseless schemes which can turn out to be financially and socially disastrous to both themselves and their families.

At one level manic patients can often be amusing and attractive and draw people to them. However, this overwhelming behaviour soon becomes exhausting and exasperating to relatives, friends and colleagues.

As their behaviour becomes increasingly out of control and disinhibited this can lead to embarrassing situations and, if this is allowed to continue, their relationships and reputation may be put in peril. If patients feel that obstacles are being put in their way they will suddenly become irritable and angry for, beneath this overactivity, they are vulnerable and sensitive to criticism and will respond to feeling thwarted with verbal abuse or even physical aggression.

Treatment

Because manic patients' behaviour is usually out of control they are likely to be at risk on several levels. On a physical level they may not find time to sleep and eat and their constant activity may produce exhaustion. On the financial and social level, their excessive spending may lead to financial difficulties where their socially disturbed behaviour may ruin their reputation amongst their families, friends and work colleagues. For example, when they are ill, manic patients often make major life decisions, such as changing their religion, partner or job, which they may later bitterly regret. It is important to get hypomanic excitement under control before it escalates into mania or plunges into depression. In order to carry out the necessary treatment it will nearly always be necessary for the patient to be admitted to hospital. Drug therapy needs to introduced right away to help reduce the psychomotor activity. Chlorpromazine and haloperidol are given in appropriate doses.

Once the manic episode is under control the psychiatrist may decide to introduce lithium carbonate to continue to control the mood. This drug has enabled considerable progress to be made in the treatment and prevention of those suffering from recurrent attacks of mania and depression.

The aftermath

The emotional and social consequence of a hypomanic attack can leave everybody around feeling devastated. As patients emerge from the episode and realise what damage they have done, they may become depressed and remorseful. This can lead to profound depression and create a different set of problems. Because such patients' behaviour is often distressing to those around them, they are likely to be the target of their wrath. Often the family routine has been upset, they may have been kept awake at night for long periods and have had to put up with all sorts of abuse and demands, which may have left everyone feeling resentful and angry.

The toll on such families can be very heavy and may well require family counselling to deal with the emotional havoc that such episodes can create. In some cases, the disruption may be so great that the partner can no longer cope with the relationship, where he or she has already experienced previous episodes of the illness and begins to fear further ones. Counselling plans need to include a medical opinion so that work can be done around the diagnosis and prognosis of the disorder, for this may be central to some of the issues which will be raised in the counselling relationship.

Hypomania can be variable and generally can be controlled with medication such as lithium and other drugs. This, of course, requires that the patients, and perhaps their families, cooperate to ensure that it is taken regularly. The family may also need assistance in identifying the first signs of the disorder, such as increased irritability, insomnia and a more expansive mood, so that patients can be referred for early help.

Assessment

Here are some of the factors which the approved social worker will need to bear in mind and consider when making a mental health assessment to decide the most appropriate course of action. Because of the behaviour already described, patients are likely to be at risk in several areas:

1   On a physical level they may feel too busy to eat, drink or sleep, and their constant activity may put them at risk through physical exhaustion and malnutrition.
2   Hypomania, if not checked, risks escalating into mania or plunging into depression.
3   On a social and financial level their extravagant and disinhibited behaviour may lead to ruin. For example, it is not uncommon for such patients to enter into senseless financial schemes or run up considerable debts through credit cards and hire purchase arrangements which can dissipate savings.

Socially uninhibited behaviour can create social damage to themselves, family, friends and colleagues and, if it is allowed to go unchecked, can destroy career and relationships. When such patients are well they may bitterly regret this and might find it difficult to undo the harm they have done.

4 If thwarted in their extravagant demands hypomanic patients can become angry and, if pressed, violent. This can create additional stresses and difficulties when family and friends want to limit their activities, and this is one reason why compulsory admission may be helpful.

Social work with the hypomanic patient

The normal personality of hypomanic patients tends to swing between extreme moods: elation to depression; exuberance to withdrawal. In a clinical sense, they are said to be cyclothymic. It may be a while before others realised that their behaviour has gone beyond the bounds of what is rational and tolerable and professional help is sought. By this time, much damage may have been done.

Although many people function at a high energy level and are often creative and successful, it is only when such behaviour oversteps the mark and patients become out of control and put themselves and others at risk that intervention is necessary. Most people who reach this level of their illness are impulsive, reckless and lacking any insight into their behaviour and need for help. Because of this it may not be possible to gain their cooperation. They may not regard themselves as ill; indeed, they may feel on top of the world. In the most severe cases they will need to be admitted to hospital, if necessary on a formal basis, to prevent further harm to themselves and others.

Functional psychoses: schizophrenia

Schizophrenia is the most severe of all the functional psychoses. The illness occurs more often in late adolescence and in early adult life but can be present in middle and old age. The term schizophrenia means 'splitting or fragmentation' of the mind and does not refer to the double 'Jekyll and Hyde' type of personality. It is perhaps best thought of as a group of related disorders which produce disorganisation of the personality. If the illness goes untreated there is a progressive disintegration which often affects judgement, emotions and behaviour. Delusions and auditory hallucinations are also often present.

In the UK the mainstream of psychiatrists use the concepts of Kurt Schneider (1959) when diagnosing schizophrenia. He identified a group of symptoms which he regards as 'first rank' in differentiating schizophrenia from other conditions. These are as follows:

1 **Thought disorders:**
   - thought insertion – the belief that thoughts are being inserted in one's mind from outside
   - thought withdrawal – the belief that thoughts are taken out of one's mind from outside
   - thought broadcasting – the belief that thoughts become known to others.

2 **Auditory hallucinations.** These are voices heard discussing one's thoughts or behaviour as they occur, like a running commentary. Such voices are often abusive, ridiculing or derogatory.
3 **Primary delusions.** The patient may suddenly develop the unshakeable belief that a particular set of events has a special meaning for him and will develop an elaborate delusional system.

In Schneider's view, if someone has one of these symptoms in the absence of organic or physical disturbance, the diagnosis points to schizophrenia.

The incidence of schizophrenia is just under 1 per cent of the population. This figure appears to be fairly even throughout the world. Schizophrenia often accounts for some 15 per cent of admissions to mental hospitals. About 45 per cent of the long-stay population in mental hospitals are schizophrenics. The illness is more common in males than females, and most cases occur before the age of 30.

The prognosis of schizophrenia is variable. For example, the speed of the onset of the illness is significant. There seems to be a more favourable prognosis where the condition develops acutely, and the previous personality was fairly well integrated. With the more insidious onset, grown slowly out of a withdrawn schizoid personality, the prognosis is poorer.

Up to approximately one-third of schizophrenic patients do not recover, except from their acute symptoms; they may be left with severe mental disabilities. In all cases of schizophrenia prompt treatment is essential to prevent further deterioration.

The general signs and symptoms of schizophrenia can be grouped under four main disorders;

- thought
- perception
- emotion
- behaviour.

Thought disorder

Many schizophrenia sufferers find it difficult to put their thoughts together in a comprehensible way. Their thinking often shows displacement or the use of associated thoughts for the correct ones.

There can be a disorder in the flow of thoughts, when patients will suddenly stop and then carry on a train of thought which may be totally unconnected with the first one. This is known as 'thought blocking'. Schneiderian first-rank symptoms of thought insertion, thought withdrawal and thought broadcasting may also be present.

Disorders of content of thought are called delusions, the most common of which are termed delusions of persecution, where patients may irrationally believe they are the subject of persecution (paranoid delusions). These are often accompanied by auditory hallucinations.

Delusions of a more bizarre nature (usually grandiose) can often be traced back to more primary delusional experience.

Other patients may believe that certain situations have a particular significance to them and that messages are being given to them (ideas of reference). They may have feelings of being controlled by outside influence (passivity feelings).

There may also be a flattening of affect in which there is a lack of emotional responsiveness.

Disorders of perception

These can take the form of hallucinations, illusions, or depersonalisation and derealisation experiences. An hallucination can be the perception that a voice or voices are talking to the person. Since a person often feels no alternative but to comply with instructions or commands from this voice or voices, this experience can lead to dangerous or unpredictable behaviour. Hallucinations arise in the senses and therefore relate to experiences of seeing, hearing, smelling, touching or tasting. Visual hallucinations however are rare in schizophrenia and if present, they are more likely to indicate the use of toxic substances such as drugs or alcohol. Illusions are the incorrect perception of real events, for example hearing a rattle and believing that there is a deadly snake somewhere nearby which will kill someone. Depersonalisation is the experience of not feeling real. Derealisation is the experience that the world itself is unreal and empty.

Disorders of emotion

In acute schizophrenia, elation, ecstasy or depression may be present. These emotions usually settle to give way to the more characteristic emotional states. The emotional reaction and mood may be inappropriate (incongruity of affect), where the patient may laugh in the wrong places, or the wrong emotion is experienced for the given situation. There may be flattening of affect, where there is lack of emotional responsiveness.

Disorders of behaviour

Withdrawal from normal social contact is a common symptom of schizophrenia. In its more extreme forms patients might withdraw into a stupor-like state (catatonia) and become motionless, mute and unresponsive to external stimuli. This state can be interrupted by sudden outbursts of excitement (catonic excitement). Frequently such patients show what is known as 'waxy flexibility' in which patients may hold their limbs in strange positions and maintain these postures for long periods of time.

These states are now rare in their more extreme manifestations but are still seen in their milder forms.

Classification of schizophrenia

It is customary to classify schizophrenia into four subgroups. This is now questioned by many psychiatrists because individuals seldom fall into such neat categories and, therefore, no hard and fast rule can be applied. However, despite the fact that there is often overlap between various groups, the different schizophrenic reactions do occur and their description remains valuable.

Simple schizophrenia

The onset occurs in adolescence and is marked by gradual withdrawal from social contacts and loss of drive. Flattening of affect and thought disorder may be present. It is said that such disorders are often undiagnosed with the result that sufferers are in danger of going untreated, leading to them drifting into vagrancy and petty crime.

Catatonic schizophrenia

The onset occurs in early life. Patients can alternate between withdrawal and muteness and exhibiting outbursts of sudden excited behaviour. This diagnosis is made less frequently in modern psychiatry, although catatonia still presents in milder forms. It is important to understand that such patients have a clear appreciation of what is happening around them and will recall lucidly when they recover.

Hebephrenic schizophrenia

Onset is usually in late adolescence. Emotional changes usually dominate the clinical picture. Such patients are usually preoccupied with pseudo-psychological and philosophical ideas; they are moody, sometimes giggly, fatuous and show characteristic incongruity of affect.

Paranoid schizophrenia

Unlike the above groups, paranoid schizophrenia has a later onset, usually between the ages of 30 and 50. Delusions of persecution and auditory hallucinations are the typical symptoms.

Unlike the other groups, the individuals' personality is usually well preserved and does not disintegrate. Delusions may be 'encapsulated' and patients behave normally until the delusional ideas bring them into conflict with society. Such patients have hypersensitive personalities and respond to most benign situations with suspicion. The prognosis is good; most cases respond favourably to neuroleptic medication.

Causes of schizophrenia

The cause of schizophrenia remains very much a matter of debate and continued investigation. No single cause is known. Evidence suggests an interplay of genetic, psychological and social factors which seem to determine the development of the illness. People who have been adopted while still young and brought up by unrelated parents have been shown to have a high risk of developing the illness. The closer someone is related to a patient with schizophrenia, the higher is the risk of developing this condition.

Among the social and psychological perspectives of possible causes those of Bateson (1956) and Laing (1960) are significant. Bateson's 'double bind' theory is concerned with the ambiguity of communication between family members and has the following factors;

1 The individual has an intense relationship with a significant other carer (usually the mother, although it can be another close person).
2 The significant carer expresses two messages when making a single statement – one message contradicting the other.
3 The individual cannot comment on the mutually contradictory messages, thus creating a confusing conflict in the individual's mind which can only find resolution in madness.

R.D. Laing's attempts to explain schizophrenia as a way of surviving the pressures of an abnormal family situation does not view schizophrenia as an illness but more as a 'behaviour label' for a certain kind of experience.

Laing argues that it is necessary to accept these experiences as valid and seek to understand them as potentially meaningful – as an existential truth. The practical effects of schizophrenia in our society are that sufferers experience a chaotic and distressing process which appears meaningless at the time and seems to destroy their capacity for full and meaningful life. Indeed, many schizophrenics are reduced by their illness into a deprived and marginal way of life.

The sociological view of drift theory has important implications for social work with the mentally ill. Some studies have been made on the nature of the relationship between social class and schizophrenia in central urban areas. The drift theory suggests that schizophrenics, as they become more disorganised and fragmented, drift into rundown areas where accommodation is cheaper and there is little social pressure on them.

Goldberg and Huxley (1980) found that the occupations of male schizophrenics tended to be less well paid and prestigious than the occupations of their fathers. In their view, this social downward mobility indicates that, as the mental illness develops, the sufferer drifts into work which is simple and often well below their educational achievement. Unless there is effective social work and medical intervention, the schizophrenic may continue to drift downwards to form the hard core of the destitute and vagrant population. Clearly, once they drift outside of the boundaries of helping agencies (fall through the care net) they can become deprived of effective treatment, being viewed merely as tramps, rather than mentally ill.

Treatment

Treatment of the schizophrenic is primarily concerned with reducing the symptoms by the use of the neuroleptic medication, which have an antipsychotic effect. By this, we mean it is successful in suppressing some of the distressing effects of the symptoms of delusions and hallucinations. These drugs were first introduced in the early 1950s and have been used extensively ever since.

However, many patients tend to stop taking medication when they leave hospital, when they begin to feel better or when they suffer side-effects. In the majority of cases stopping medication leads to relapse to their former symptoms.

Social workers must be aware of the effects and possible side-effects of these drugs and be able to describe these to patients and to liaise effectively with other professionals in the management of patients' medication. Default in medication is so common in schizophrenia that long-acting neuroleptic injections have been developed to cope with the problem. Depixol and Modecate are given to the patient by community psychiatric nurses (CPNs) in the form of intramuscular injections at regular intervals in the patient's home or at an outpatients clinic.

Many of the drugs mentioned above can have side-effects. Drugs taken in large doses can produce drowsiness, tremor, restlessness, facial grimaces, protrusion of the tongue and chewing movements (tardive dyskinesia) and also symptoms mimicking Parkinson's disease, such as mask-like faces. Anti-Parkinson symptom drugs, such as procyclidine, may be given to counteract these unpleasant side-effects.

Drug therapy

Major tranquillisers (neuroleptics)

Neuroleptics form the major tranquillisers and are used in the treatment of schizophrenia, hypomania and other mental disorders. Neuroleptic drugs have been used for over 40 years; they have stood the test of time in treating some of the gross behaviour of psychotic disturbance.

Phenothiazines

Phenothiazines are a subgroup which includes the standard drugs such as Largactil and Stelazine. These have an antipsychotic effect in the sense that they calm the patient and reduce much of the distress caused by the positive symptoms of auditory hallucinations and delusions. Psychiatrists question whether these drugs reverse the psychotic process or whether they simply act by suppressing the psychotic symptoms and anxiety. All these drugs seem to be effective in diminishing the emotional response to both the internal and external stimuli.

Since the phenothiazine drugs were first developed in the early 1950s, other types have been developed from the same chemical family and include Melleril, Fentazin and Sparine. It is often a matter of clinical judgement which particular drugs are used.

Butyrophenones

These drugs are more potent than the above tranquillisers and are primarily used to act on the dopamine receptors in the brain in order to slow down psychomotor activity. Haloperidol is the most popular drug in this group. However, this drug is slowly excreted from the body, and its cumulative effect can soon produce toxicity. It is therefore usually given in smaller doses to reduce the risk of toxic effects. The side-effects from this group tend to be greater than those found in phenothiazines.

Minor tranquillisers (anxiolytics)

Anxiolytics are the minor tranquillisers and, because they have attracted much publicity because of their abuse, they have become household names. They include drugs such as Valium and Librium which, when used carefully, are effective in reducing much of the anxiety associated with the psycho-neuroses and sometimes in the withdrawal symptoms of alcoholism. Unlike the major tranquillisers, the side-effects from this group of drugs are minimal. However, there is growing evidence that many people become dependent on these drugs and, if they stop taking them suddenly, they do suffer from withdrawal symptoms which can include symptoms of sleeplessness, acute panic and depression.

It should be stressed that all drugs potentate the effects with alcohol.

Sedatives

As the name suggests, these drugs sedate and are primarily used in the treatment of insomnia. Sleep disturbance is a common symptom of many psychiatric conditions, particularly depression, mania, schizophrenia and other disorders where there is marked increase in anxiety.

Barbiturates were the most frequently prescribed group of sedatives until they were found to have an addictive effect. Their use became open to abuse, causing numerous overdose fatalities.

These drugs have now been replaced in favour of the safer and less addictive benzodiazepine group of drugs. Hypnotic drugs are useful in helping induce sleep, but do not affect the underlying cause of sleep disturbance.

Antidepressant medication

Antidepressant medication has made possible a major breakthrough in the treatment of depression. Such drugs can be divided into two main groups – the tricyclics and the monoamine oxidase inhibitors (MAOIs).

Before the introduction of MAOIs, amphetamines or so-called 'pep pills' were commonly used to treat clinical depression. These drugs produced rapid dependence, and doses had to be increased to achieve the desired effect. Although they temporarily lifted the patient's mood they did not address the basic cause of the depressive illness, with the result that the patient was often left feeling flat, empty and more depressed. In large doses amphetamines induced terrifying feelings of persecution, sometimes in the form of visual hallucination. This syndrome came to be known as the 'horrors' – a form of paranoid psychosis. These drugs are no longer used in the treatment of depression and have been replaced by the groups described below.

Tricyclics

Unlike the neuroleptics and sedatives, tricyclics do not affect the mood right away. The improvement is usually felt by the patient over a period of time, usually between seven and 21 days after treatment has commenced. These drugs must therefore be taken for the full period before it is certain they are going to work.

Studies have shown that this group of drugs is the safest and most effective antidepressant medication. About two-thirds of depressed patients respond and improve on them. Patients who do best are those who suffer from clear-cut depressive illness with restlessness and anxiety. Because these drugs contain a compound with a pronounced sedative effect (chemically they are related to the neuroleptics) a dose can often be taken at night to help produce a good night's sleep.

Antidepressant medication has considerably reduced the need for electroconvulsive therapy. Tricyclics given simultaneously with ECT can often reduce the number of ECT treatments required.

It is also interesting to note that this kind of medication has no effect in elevating the mood of 'normal' people. It is only effective where there is a depressive mood disorder. In other words, tricyclics do not act as euphoriants like amphetamines which have a more direct stimulating effect on the central nervous system.

Lithium carbonate

Lithium carbonate is a simple substance which is sometimes successfully used in the short- and long-term treatment of affective disorders. It has also been shown to prevent, or substantially reduce, manic and depressive episodes where there is a recurrence of these mood swings. Patients who seem to benefit most are those who have suffered a manic depressive illness and who have experienced about three episodes during the previous five years. Three principal factors are crucial when considering such treatment:

1 the severity of the affective disorder;
2 the wishes of the patient;
3 the patient's reliability in taking regular medication.

This third point is very important for patients must attend hospital or clinic regularly for blood tests. A high degree of cooperation is necessary for treatment to be effective.

Because affective disorder seems to be a lifelong illness, treatment must be planned accordingly. Lithium carbonate would seem to be the most appropriate way of managing the illness once the patient's confidence has been established.

Drug side-effects

Neuroleptic medication

The phenothiazine group of drugs has become the standard medication for the treatment of schizophrenia. They are also used in other major psychotic disorders and have brought considerable relief to the sufferers. These drugs do, however, produce unwanted side-effects – known as extrapyramidal symptoms – and these can be listed under the following four groups.

Pseudo Parkinsonism This mimics some of the signs and symptoms of Parkinson's disease. The patient develops a mask-like facial expression, tremor of the hands and a general stiffening of the limbs.

Akathisia This condition is marked by restlessness where the patient is unable to keep still, fidgets, tends to shuffle and rocks his or her body backwards and forwards.

Acute dyskinesia These are more acute reactions. Oculogyric crisis is the most common. It starts with a fixed stare, then the eyes turn upwards and this is followed by great tension in the neck and opening of the mouth. This is a most alarming sight and can last a few hours before subsiding spontaneously.

Other dyskinesic reactions can affect the trunk and limbs, producing grotesque postures or writhing movements. All these reactions are extremely distressing both to the patient and the onlooker.

Chronic tardive dyskinesia This is characterised by continuous chewing movements, rolling the head, and frequently sticking out the tongue as if to lick the lips. There can be certain changes in a person's posture. These symptoms can persist even after the neuroleptic medication has been stopped. The patient might also complain of a dry mouth, blurred vision and weight gain, although the latter symptom may be the result of the fact that phenothiazine can stimulate the appetite.

Antidepressant medication

Like other drug groups, antidepressant medication can produce unwanted side-effects although, in the case of tricyclics, they are less severe. These include hypotension (reduced blood pressure), constipation, urinary delay, blurred vision and, in very rare cases, hypomania. This latter effect is usually found in patients who are prone to recurrent mood disorders.

Depot injections

There are many patients who need to take medication on a regular basis, over long periods of time, while others may need to take it for the rest of their lives. Depot injections are long-acting slow-releasing neuroleptic drugs which are given at regular intervals, usually between two to four weeks, the particular dose depending on individual needs. This method of administering medication has been shown to be more reliable and effective than oral medication.

Some patients stop taking their medication for a number of reasons, usually perhaps because they feel better and no longer feel the need to continue taking tablets. Others may find the side-effects too distressing and then fail to persevere with them. Yet other patients may be too confused, lack insight or forget to take them due to the nature of their illness. Non-compliance with medication is the most common cause of relapse and need for re-admission to hospital in schizophrenics. The treatment of schizophrenia involves a complex interaction between medication and the psychosocial factors in the patient's life. For example, it has been shown that neuroleptics reduce the risk of relapse.

Depot injections come in various forms. Depixol-Modecate is the most widely used. The injections are administered intramuscularly in the patient's buttock, producing a store of the drug in the body. By drawing on this store gradually a certain level of the drug is sustained in the blood so that the brain is able to extend control over the symptoms for a period of two to four weeks.

Depot injections are usually given to the patient at home or in special outpatient clinics by the community psychiatric nurse. The regular contact between the CPN and the patient also offers the opportunity to monitor the patient's general progress.

Electroconvulsive therapy (ECT)

Some information on the historical development and mode of action of ECT is given here in the hope that this will give workers a better understanding of this often controversial form of treatment. It is also hoped that this might dispel some of the misconceptions surrounding this type of therapy.

In the 1920s it was observed that some epileptics who also suffered from schizophrenia seemed to improve following an epileptic seizure. Often the disorder of thought and mood would temporarily clear. This prompted some workers to postulate that schizophrenia and epilepsy were biologically antagonistic. (This later proved to be a mistaken belief.) Such a view encouraged others to experiment with ways of artificially inducing epileptic fits in schizophrenics.

Meduna, in 1933, began testing the ability of chemical substances such as camphor and, later, cardizol to produce seizures. Patients using these substances showed some improvement. However, this method was extremely crude and the fits produced were uncontrolled and difficult to terminate, which made such treatment hazardous.

It was not until Cerlette and Bini introduced an electrical method of introducing convulsions in 1938 that a more universal interest grew. This method used bitemporal electrodes which passed an electrical current through the brain, rendering the patient unconscious and producing a *grand mal* seizure. This technique enabled the doctor, for the first time, to exercise a greater control over its duration and extent.

The most dangerous complications resulting from this method were fractures and dislocations of bones resulting from the violence of the fit. ECT was first introduced into the UK in 1940. An important modification was made in 1941 when curare was introduced to paralyse the patient's muscles during treatment. This was given without a general anaesthetic but did reduce the above complications. In the 1950s short-acting anaesthetics were given together with muscle relaxants, rendering the patient unconscious and preventing him or her from consciously experiencing the frightening respiratory paralysis and the general fear associated with the treatment.

Anaesthesia was only given in sufficient quantity to ensure an adequate convulsion (that is, a *grand mal* epileptic fit). It was the quality of the fit which appeared crucial to the effectiveness of ECT.

From its crude origins ECT was becoming more humane and sophisticated and, with the help of a competent anaesthetist, it became a remarkably safe treatment. Such technical advances were not, however, matched by an understanding of how the treatment worked, and many remained opposed to its use.

Epileptic seizures have always been the subject of fear and stigma to the general public. To many, artificially inducing such seizures seems denigrating and brutal.

Since the introduction of antidepressant medication, the use of ECT has been substantially reduced. It is now used sparingly, often only in those cases where medication has failed to bring relief and only for specific disorders. These can be summarised as severely depressed patients, who suffer from endogenous depression in which they experience mental retardation, nihilistic delusions, agitation, life-threatening weight loss and suicidal thoughts. Some authorities also believe it to be of benefit in mania, some schizophrenic patients and in the treatment of puerperal psychoses.

ECT is customarily given two or three times per week. Since memory disturbance has been minimised it can now be given more frequently, although this is seldom done. Many respond well to five treatments but others may require more. If improvements do not occur after seven convulsions it is rarely advisable to continue.

The issue of brain damage as a result of ECT remains debatable. Clearly, the treatment interferes with brain function as is evidenced by resulting confusion and memory disturbances. There is, however, no evidence to suggest that structural brain damage occurs. Objective tests have shown that memory disturbance following treatment disappears after one month. It might be helpful if we look at the step-by-step medical procedure adopted for the administration of ECT.

Mode of treatment

Before ECT is administered, a thorough medical examination is made to ensure that the patient is fit enough to undergo the treatment. This is normal procedure when a general anaesthetic is given. Although ECT can be given on an outpatient basis, it is better to carry it out on an inpatient so that observation may be made before and after treatment.

Treatment is usually conveniently given in the morning, when the patient should not eat or drink anything. Half an hour before the treatment, an injection or premedication of atropine and a tranquilliser is given. The former helps prevent salivation and vomiting and the tranquilliser allays anxiety. Before ECT treatment is administered the patient is seen by the anaesthetist who gives an intravenous injection of a short-acting anaesia (thiopentone) and a muscle relaxant. The psychiatrist then places the unilateral electrodes either side of the patient's head and a fit is then induced by an electric current. The convulsion usually occurs immediately and lasts about 30 to 40 seconds. The patient is given oxygen by the anaesthetist until spontaneous respiration is re-established. He or she is then laid on his or her side until consciousness is regained between five to 15 minutes later. On recovery, the patient may be confused and suffer from memory disturbance. This is a temporary phase, however, and passes after a short period of time.

The mechanism by which ECT works is not yet fully understood; indeed, it remains a mystery. The improvement in the patient's mood is not so much related to the amount of electric current passed as to the extent of the fit that is induced. ECT is given in a course and the amount of treatment is largely determined by the results achieved at each session.

Psychosurgery (leucotomy)

Eqas Moniz, a Portuguese surgeon, developed the first leucotomy operation in 1936, and this became the standard practice until the 1950s when it fell into disrepute because of the high number of side-effects.

The operation (which literally means cutting the white matter) consists of drilling two burr holes, one on each side of the frontal part of the skull. A knife known as a leucotome is then used to sever and divide the white fibre tracts between the frontal lobes and the hypothalamus parts of the brain. The pathway is responsible for the regulation of emotional responses and tension.

Prefrontal leucotomies were performed on a large number of patients with a wide range of mental disorders. The early claims that the operation could cure symptoms of schizophrenia and chronic depression soon lost ground, however, for many patients developed side-effects which were often worse than their original disorder. They included an increase in apathy, inertia, loss of initiative and drive. Many were reduced to vegetable-like existence with flat emotional response, loss of judgement and deterioration of social behaviour. Others developed epilepsy and became incontinent.

During the 1960s the operation was modified (bimedial or rostral) and seemed to incur a lower incidence of side-effects and complications. In the 1970s the operation underwent further developments and the stereotactic leucotomy was introduced. In this operation small areas of the brain could be destroyed with great accuracy and on a specific site and, again, claims were made that it had further reduced side-effects.

Those who are referred for psychosurgery must have been treated extensively with all other forms of treatment without effect. It seems to benefit the following disorders:

- longstanding and severe obsessional states
- chronic depression
- certain schizophrenic conditions
- intractable severe pain.

Hormonal implant treatment

Hormonal implants are used primarily in the treatment of sexual offenders when efforts to administer the hormones orally have proven unreliable. The effect of the treatment is to reduce the male libido to the point of impotence. Since 1963 this treatment has been carried out on sexual offenders where the criteria consist of subjective certainty of reconviction if no help is given, that the individual's history suggests reconviction, and that the IQ is too low, or there is limited capacity to verbalise difficulties, making the person unsuitable for psychotherapy.

Hormonal implant treatment is carried out mainly in prison settings where, in most cases, the prisoner is serving a sentence for sexual assault on children. Due to the highly controversial nature of the treatment, the Mental Health Act 1983 provides stringent safeguards to protect patients' and prisoners' rights. Legal requirements concerning ECT, psychosurgery and hormonal implant treatment are dealt with in Chapter 1.

Consent to treatment

The legal position of a detained mental patient concerning consent to, or refusal of, treatment is clarified under Part IV of the Mental Health Act 1983. Set out below are the main provisions as they apply to social workers and their clients.

Exclusions from the Act: common law rights

Part IV of the Act does not apply to informal patients, nor to those detained under short-term orders (Sections 4 and 136 are the most relevant exclusions for social workers), nor to guardianship patients. Patients who are so excluded have the same rights to refuse treatment as does any patient admitted to a general hospital with a physical disorder. This is a right under common law. Where such patients cannot give consent but are not withholding consent (e.g. a demented patient), and the situation is not an emergency, the nearest relative should be approached for consent. If there is no nearest relative, a court order should be considered.

Under common law medical treatment without consent may be given in an emergency or in cases of necessity. Necessity is not defined in law, but it mainly covers instances of unconsciousness, accidents and life-saving measures. In most cases the responsibility for taking such decisions lies with the doctor.

Where Part IV applies

As we have said, this includes patients compulsorily admitted for 28 days or longer, that is, Sections 2 and 3. The Act sets out three categories of medical treatment: Category 1, psychosurgery and sex hormone implant treatment; Category 2, medication after it has been administered for three months, and ECT; Category 3, any other treatment for mental disorder administered under the direction of the responsible medical officer.

Category 1: psychosurgery and sex hormone implant treatment
The statutory authority for this is Section 57. Under this section, treatment cannot be given unless the patient consents *and a second opinion agrees*: this consent must be confirmed by a doctor other than the responsible medical officer and also two other non-medical persons, all appointed by the Mental Health Act Commission. Before issuing a certificate to proceed with the treatment the doctor must consult two other people who have been concerned with the patient's treatment, one a nurse and the other neither a nurse nor a doctor.

Section 57 also applies to informal patients, in view of the potentially irreversible nature of the treatment.

Category 2: medication after it has been administered for three months and ECT
The statutory authority for this is Section 58. Under this section treatment cannot be given unless the patient agrees, or a second opinion agrees. The responsible medical officer or a doctor appointed by the Mental Health Act Commission must certify in writing that the patient is capable of comprehending what the treatment is, its effects and purpose; and has consented to it. Where consent from the patient is not given, then a doctor appointed by the commission (not the responsible medical officer) must certify in writing that the patient is not capable of comprehending the treatment, or has not consented to it, but that 'having regard to the likelihood of it alleviating or preventing a deterioration of his condition, the treatment should be given'.

Before issuing the certificate to proceed with treatment the independent doctor must consult two other people who have been professionally concerned with the patient's medical treatment – one a nurse, the other neither a nurse nor a doctor.

Withdrawal of consent
Section 60 provides that a patient can withdraw his consent to treatment at any time, except for cases of emergency. This is also a basic right under common law.

Category 3: any other treatment
This can range from nursing to psychoanalysis, and includes most of the day-to-day therapeutic activities within hospital. The patient can be treated without consent or a second opinion.

Urgent treatment
Under Section 62 any treatment to which Part IV of the Act applies can be administered without the need for consent or a second opinion if it is urgent. This means that it is necessary to save the patient's life, is not irreversible, and is

immediately necessary to prevent a serious deterioration in the patient's condition, or prevent harm to others.

The Bournewood example

'L' was an adult with autism. He was admitted voluntarily to Bournewood at the age of 14, then at the age of 45 had moved to live with Mr and Mrs E, but continued attendance at a day centre once a week. Whilst there one day he became agitated and his carers could not be contacted. He was taken to the accident and emergency department at Bournewood. His agitation increased and he was seen by a psychiatrist. L was then voluntarily admitted to a behavioural unit. A writ of habeas corpus and damages for false imprisonment were refused by the High Court. The Court of Appeal reversed this decision on appeal. It was held that L had been detained and that the Mental Health Act 1983 required mentally incapacitated patients to be admitted under its provisions dealing with compulsory admission and that thus L had been unlawfully detained. An appeal was made to the House of Lords. (R v Bournewood Community and Mental Health NHS Trust [1983] 3 All ER 289), the House of Lords allowed the appeal. They ruled that a mentally disordered person lacking any capacity to consent could be admitted to hospital as an informal patient under s.131 (1) of the Mental Health Act 1983 'Informal admission of patients', which states:

Nothing in this Act shall be construed as preventing a patient who requires treatment for mental disorder from being admitted to any hospital or nursing home in pursuance of arrangements made in that behalf and without application, order or direction rendering him liable to be detained under this Act, or from remaining in any hospital or mental nursing home in pursuance of such arrangements after he has ceased to be liable so to be detained. (MHA, Jones 1996, p. 338)

The principle adopted here was the common law doctrine of necessity. The circumstances of the Bournewood case rightly urge ASWs and others concerned with the long term care and treatment of people who are not able to give informed consent to be vigilant about the human rights of those in their charge.

Psychotherapy

Psychotherapy may broadly be defined as any psychological treatment which uses verbal communication to understand and influence the patient's attitudes and behaviour. Using this definition, psychotherapy is practised by many social workers in varying degrees of intensity, ranging from brief focused and irregular contact to more regular and formally structured sessions over a period of time.

Psychotherapy can be divided into the following types.

1   individual psychotherapy:

  - supportive
  - intensive
  - psychoanalysis

2   group psychotherapy
3   marital and family therapy
4   behaviour therapy

Individual psychotherapy

Supportive psychotherapy

This is perhaps the most widely used type of psychotherapy used in psychiatry. It entails the following techniques which have much in common with the social casework process.

1   **Ventilation.** This offers the patient the opportunity to express problems both in the 'here and now' and those which have occurred in the past.
2   **Clarification.** Here problems are discussed and the therapist helps the patient understand how the past may be affecting his or her present behaviour.
3   **Abreaction.** This process enables the patient to express highly charged emotions within the safety of the therapeutic relationship. This usually includes feelings of rage, resentment, anxiety and grief.
4   **Suppression.** The therapist is more authoritarian in this role and often uses a more directive approach – that is, he or she gives advice, and uses persuasion and suggestion.

Intensive psychotherapy

This method is more structured and entails greater skills in dealing with the unconscious processes. The main body of theory is based on Freud, Klein and Jung and uses the central concept of transference to understand unconscious motivation. This type of therapy is practised by qualified psychotherapists who, in addition to having a basic qualification in, say, social work or psychology, will have undergone full psychotherapy training which has included their own personal analysis as part of the process. This will have helped the therapist deal with the problems in his or her own make-up so that they do not harmfully interfere with the objectivity and effectiveness of the therapeutic relationship. In contrast to supportive psychotherapy, the patient is usually seen on a regular basis, for an hour several times a week, over a period of time.

In intensive psychotherapy the therapist takes on a more objective role, using the phenomenon known as transference in which the patient transfers emotions he has towards important figures in his past – for example, his mother and father – towards the therapist. During the treatment, the patient begins to re-experience those feelings and conflicts which may have shaped his or her present difficulties.

The analysis of the transference relationship is crucial to understanding and reconstructing the patient's unconscious neurosis so that it can be faced and worked through in the relationship with the psychotherapist. The constant repetition of these early patterns of experience, and the subsequent interpretation of them, eventually brings conviction, insight and change into how the patient deals with his or her problems. Most patients who are referred for this type of psychotherapy suffer from personality difficulties – psycho-neuroses – which prevent them from making satisfactory relationships. This form of psychotherapy is not generally regarded as being suitable for psychotic conditions.

Clearly, such treatment is time-consuming and costly and, because it is not always available on the National Health Service, much will depend on the local services in a particular area, the severity of the disorder and whether alternative methods of treatment are available. Psychotherapy requires considerable cooperation in terms of time and effort and those who are referred for this type of therapy must fulfil fairly rigorous criteria. They need, for example, to be well motivated, have the ability to verbalise and have the necessary ego strength to bear the pain of insight and change.

Because psychotherapy is not readily available on the NHS, many psychotherapists practise privately and set their fees on a sliding scale to help less well off patients afford the treatment. The British Confederation of Psychotherapists (BCP) and the United Kingdom Council for Psychotherapy (UKCP) both hold registers of psychotherapists who subscribe to their respective codes of ethics. Psychotherapeutic training bodies may accept patients on reduced fees.

Psychoanalysis

Psychoanalysis is the technique of investigation and therapy devised by

Freud for the treatment of neurosis and personality disorders. Unlike the psychotherapy just described it entails seeing the patient five times a week over a period of years. The term 'psychoanalysis' is widely used but often in an inexact sense. Strictly speaking, it should only be used to describe orthodox analysis which is a process practised by a psychoanalyst – that is, a medical or layperson who has fulfilled the training requirements of the British Psychoanalytical Society and has undergone a minimum period of personal analysis as part of his or her training. Although both individual and group psychotherapy may use Freudian theory they should not be confused with psychoanalysis. Jung and Adler, both pupils of Freud, broke away and founded their own methods of therapy. These are called analytical psychotherapy and individual psychology, respectively.

Patients undertaking psychoanalysis present a wide range of personality difficulties, ranging from neurotic phobias to delinquent behaviour. Many have had other forms of psychiatric treatment. Before clinical criteria are considered patients must be able to afford the time and money, for it is not available on the NHS. The Institute of Psychoanalysis in London accepts some patients on a reduced fee.

Most analyses are conducted on a private basis and, like private psychotherapy, fees are usually charged on a sliding scale depending on the patient's financial circumstances.

Group psychotherapy

Unlike individual psychotherapy, the main focus of interest in group psychotherapy is the interrelationships within the group. Individual problems are shared and members can often see their personal difficulties reflected in the relationships within the group. Each member is then able to contribute his or her comments, and the therapist's role is to interpret the problems that invariably arise in the group.

In many ways, this kind of therapy has great advantages over individual psychotherapy for those with marked social and interpersonal difficulties. Indeed, some workers would argue that this ought to be the treatment of choice for those patients whose main problems centre around communication and social relationships. Many of the basic concepts of psychoanalytical theory and a whole body of theoretical knowledge about group work has evolved in the understanding of group processes. It is the group therapist's role to interpret resistant and defensive behaviour and thereby facilitate interaction. Group therapy sessions are usually held once or twice weekly on an outpatient basis and last for about one and a half hours. Group therapy can continue over a period of years depending on the needs and progress of individual patients.

Most psychiatric settings practise group work and often these are modified versions of group psychotherapy to help patients develop the capacity to gain confidence and discuss problems with others.

Marital and family therapy

A great deal has been written about marital and family therapy and social workers and psychotherapists on both sides of the Atlantic display much interest in it. It is an area of constant development and growth. In this section we do not aspire to a new construction, but present an overview of the more common approaches that currently exist.

It was Jung who first alluded to family-centred therapeutic intervention, in relation to childhood disturbances. He stated quite clearly that childhood disturbances pointed to underlying conflicts in the marital relationship of the parents and that, unless these were resolved, the child could not fully resolve his or her difficulties.

Marriage and mental health

A wide range of evidence, particularly from the USA, has highlighted the relationship between mental health and marriage. Married people tend to have lower rates of hospitalisation, lower rates of outpatient treatment as well as lower rates of alcoholism and suicide. Married people tend to live longer than the unmarried.

In recent years, sociologists have mounted a critique of the family, noting its historical associations with property rights, the state and male and female hierarchical roles.

Nowadays, the concept of 'family' is increasingly open to question, and family forms vary between cultures. According to research by the Joseph Rowntree Foundation (July 1998), various children's perspectives on families show some correlation: 'From children's point of view, love, care and mutual respect and support were the key characteristics of family.' Moreover, the past decade has seen the proportion of people living together as married couples decrease, whilst cohabitation has increased: 'In common with the United Kingdom, most European Union (EU) countries have seen a decline in marriage rates since 1985' (*Social Trends*, 1998: 50). During this period, divorce rates have increased: 'The number of divorces involving couples with children aged under 16 in England and Wales peaked at 95 thousand' (ibid.: 51). A research review conducted by Rowntree of over 200 reports (June 1998) indicates that children of separated families have a higher probability of a range of social problems persisting into adulthood, but that such problems can be mitigated by access to sufficient financial resources, emotional consistency and the maintainance of positive relations with both parents.

There may be positive indications, therefore, for family therapy to be considered in parental relationships where there is divorce, separation, discord or disharmony.

Theoretical approaches to family therapy

As with any form of therapeutic intervention there are as many approaches to family therapy as there are family therapists. Nevertheless there are some essential concepts that inform and help create the various 'schools' of family therapy. Training in family therapy has rightly become increasingly rigorous since the first edition of this book, so, although some key concepts are sketched out below, interested readers are referred to the 'References and further reading' at the end of this book for direct source material.

Psychoanalytic approaches

Practice stemming from this model tends to use group psychotherapeutic methods within a framework of human development and group interaction seen from a psychoanalytic perspective. Group analysts such as Foulkes (1964, 1975) and Bion (1961, 1967) generated much original work in the area of group psychotherapy. Skynner (1976) synthesised a number of analytic approaches into a group application suitable for work with families.

Structural approaches

Structuralists view the family as a living structure in which systems and subsystems exist and which are negotiated between family members. Therapeutic intervention aims at helping the family redefine these structures. Theoretically this reallocates power and creates more flexible roles and boundaries. Salvadore Minuchin (1974) was perhaps a key exponent of this methodology.

Solution-focused approaches

Solution-focused approaches concentrate on the solution not the problem. For solution-focused therapists, family therapy has for too long addressed the 'problem' rather than empowered families (or individuals) to find their own solutions. Solution-focused work aims to help people uncover the goals which they wish to achieve in their lives, sometimes by asking the 'miracle' question – that is, if a miracle happened overnight, how would you know, when you awoke the next day, that the miracle had happened? What would be different about your world?' – and then trying to uncover what the person might do to achieve steps towards that state. In the UK, George, Iveson and Ratner (1990) and in the USA, De Shazer (1985) are the key proponents of this approach.

Communication approaches

This approach views difficulties within the family equlibrium as arising from difficulties in communication in that communications are either faulty, unclear or expressed in the form of a 'double bind'. The therapist's task is to help communication pass in a more clear and direct way.

In the USA proponents of this approach have been the Palo Alto Group (Bateson *et al.*, 1956) and Satir (1964). In the UK Laing and Esterson (1966) developed this approach.

Behavioural approaches

Behaviour modification techniques have been used by some family therapists as an approach to therapy. This focuses on the symptoms of the difficulty. In marital therapy one simple example of this would be where the husband agrees to empty the dustbins, while the wife in response agrees to make the tea more often.

A practical approach to family therapy

We have given above some of the main strands of theory as they apply to family therapy. We would emphasise, however, that these need not be rigid approaches and, indeed, sometimes a combination of approaches or an integrative model is used. In addition, the personality of the therapist – whether he or she is active or passive, controlling or enabling, noisy or silent – will play a great part in the therapeutic process, perhaps more than dogmatic technique. It is therefore important for the therapist to be aware of his or her own personality and the effect the family is having on him or her and, conversely, the effect that this personality is having on the family. The therapist's choice of approach will give him or her clear information about the feelings and pressure which exist within the family.

General considerations   Any form of family therapy will need to address the following issues.

1   **Venue**. This is usually the clinician's office or consulting room.

2   **Whom to invite.** Some family therapists feel that all family members should attend; others that only those that dwell under the same roof should be present. Certainly the more members that attend the clearer will be the dynamics that emerge.
3   **Purpose.** The therapist will need to demonstrate a belief that the meeting is valuable to offer and must make the purpose of the meeting quite clear. Will the family be expected to sit and talk? Might they be expected to take part in 'action' sessions such as sculpting or psychodrama.*
4   **Frequency.** Weekly? Fortnightly? Monthly? This needs to be clarified with the family. Many experienced therapists feel that some space needs to be left between meetings to give the family time to digest the contents of the sessions. Skynner (1976) suggests a three weekly gap between sessions.
5   **Duration.** Weeks? Months? Years? This cannot be determined at the outset. An initial contract of, say, six meetings may be helpful, reviewable at the last session, or before, if need be.
6   **To conduct the therapy alone or with a co-therapist.** Increasingly, family therapy sessions are led by two therapists so that a wider range of interventions is made possible.

In many child guidance clinics, the use of one-way screens and videos are now common practice, with observers taking an advisory role as the sessions take place.

Behavioural therapy

Several behaviour therapy techniques have been developed to treat a wide range of psychiatric disorders and these are summarised below. As this approach derives from clinical psychological research, most of those involved in therapy and supervision are clinical psychologists. However, other people who are involved in the daily life of the patient may also play a major role in the treatment; these can include nurse, parent, teacher and social worker.

Desensitisation (reciprocal inhibition)

This model was first employed by Joseph Wolpe (1958) with patients suffering from anxiety-related problems. He found that, if patients were gradually exposed to objects or situations which they feared, whilst at the same time

---

* Family sculpting is a technique where a family member will put others into the positions, physically and in terms of proximity, that they feel best describe the situation in the household. 'Psychodrama' is the acting out of some important life event, in order to give participants more understanding of the event, its causes and effects.

engaged in pleasant activity (in Wolpe's case, he taught them deep muscle relaxation), this tended to inhibit anxiety.

Wolpe encouraged his patients first to imagine the objects and situations which aroused their fear. Patients were then given a graded series of anxiety-inducing situations, from the least to the most disturbing. As the sessions progressed, patients gradually began to tolerate the most disturbing situations as they ascended the hierarchy, first in their imaginations and then in real-life situations.

The patient's ability to experience these stressful events in the imagination was often followed by diminished anxiety when faced with them in real life. This therapy is most successful if there is a specific, clearly defined fear or impulse – for example, a phobia of insects or of flying. It is not so effective with more generalised fears such as agoraphobia.

Implosive therapy (flooding)

While systematic desensitisation exposes patients to their fears gradually, implosive therapy involves a more immediate exposure to the phobic situation. With this technique patients are encouraged to imagine themselves in the most anxiety-provoking situation possible on the grounds that the anxiety condition will be extinguished if the patient can be prevented from avoiding or escaping from the causal situation. The therapist continues to provide additional images and cues to help maximise the patient's anxiety. Usually, the treatment session ends when the patient imagines the worst situations, all the therapist's efforts to increase the patient's anxiety cease, and the patient's anxiety level falls.

With the flooding technique, the therapist takes the patient to real-life phobic situations but does not make any effort to increase the stimulus further. With each technique the session must continue until the anxiety level falls, otherwise no extinction will take place.

Assertion training

In social situations some people find it difficult to ask for something which is their due. This is sometimes now referred to as 'social phobia'. Many others experience untold misery because they find social contact embarrassing and difficult, and eventually withdraw and lead isolated lives. These are some of the clients who might benefit from assertion therapy.

Clients are encouraged to express their feelings to others in a gradual way, thereby making each new situation less and less frightening. The result of such an approach has a good deal in common with that described in the desensitisation approach above. Inhibited individuals are helped to take a bolder attitude towards social situations, taking risks and gradually learning to enjoy self-expression without continually fearing the rejection of others.

Operant conditioning

Following the work of Skinner (1953), this type of treatment was first introduced in the USA in the early 1950s. The technique involves attempting to shape behaviour by means of rewards and punishments and was initially directed at work with severely disturbed patients in mental hospitals.

Perhaps the best known and most extensive approach is the token economy system. Applications throughout the 1960s in the USA indicated how the behaviour of extremely regressed patients could be changed or modified by this approach. Patients were given rewards for desired behaviour: for example, for good self-care in terms of making their own beds and keeping themselves clean. These rewards took the form of plastic tokens which could later be exchanged for special privileges or extra visits to the canteen to buy chocolate and so on. The rewarding of desired behaviour and the ignoring or penalising of undesired behaviour increased the incidence of the former and reduced that of the latter.

It was shown that this simple principle not only reduced antisocial behaviour on the ward but also increased staff morale as a result of their creative involvement.

This behaviour approach is now used in the everyday management of rehabilitation wards of mental hospitals in the UK. Modification of the most difficult antisocial aspects of patients' behaviour enables them to become more acceptable to others and eases their adjustment into the community on discharge.

3 Severe and enduring mental illness

Introduction

Those suffering from severe and enduring mental health problems will form the main group of service users who will require the continuing care of the psychiatric services. The *Building Bridges* document, issued by the Department of Health, pinpointed three principal elements of severe mental illness. These are disability, diagnosis and duration with the addition of two further aspects, safety and the need for informal and formal care.

Before users can be seriously considered to be suffering from enduring mental illness it must have persisted for at least one year, and many will have a range of diagnoses which may include severe affective and neurotic disorders and dementia. The largest group will be those suffering from schizophrenia, who will have the positive symptoms of hallucinations, delusions and thought disorder.

Mental illness is rarely an isolated event. In some it may never return after the first episode; with others, it is likely to return at some point; and for yet others it may reoccur and persist throughout their lives. It is with this latter group that we will be concerned in this chapter.

Many of these patients may go on to suffer the negative symptoms, such as reduced emotional responsiveness, lack of concentration and energy, and social withdrawal. These symptoms usually lead to chaotic and neglectful behaviour and make survival in the community difficult to sustain. According to Leff (1997) about a quarter of patients recover completely from the first episode and do not suffer a recurrence for at least five years. Some patients remain symptom-free for many years and live relatively normal lives in the community.

Studies by the World Health Organization show that in developing world cultures the outcome is even better than this. Nearly half of the patients recover and do not relapse for several years. Reasons for this are not fully understood but may be related to tolerant and accepting family and social structures which become fragmented in industrialised cultures.

From hospital to community care

In the past, many of these service users would have formed the core of the long-stay mental hospital population. In this setting care would have been given and monitored with relative ease because all the resources would have been available under one roof. Now that the care is delivered in the community users are faced with a complex range of services – health, social services, DSS and housing. This network of services would perplex most of us but the users and their carers find it particularly difficult to access such services. Indeed, despite careful planning and communication, some users fall through the net of the psychiatric services and do not receive the help they need. In recent years there have been a number of incidents of this kind, often with tragic consequences. It has been these high-profile cases which have drawn public and professional concern and have led to the new changes in the law relating to mental health.

This new legislation has identified a specific group of users who are most at risk to themselves and others and is concerned that they receive adequate care, support and supervision and to assist them from falling through the care net.

Needs

The needs of those experiencing enduring mental health problems have been dealt with in a number of studies (Mann and Cree, 1976; Wing and Brown, 1970; Kuipers *et al.*, 1989). All these authors have recognised that users suffer from multiple disadvantages, ranging from the positive symptoms to the negative symptoms and secondary disabilities which often impair their ability to function effectively in the community. Users often have a limited range of survival and social skills, such as self-care, domestic and interpersonal skills, and, in the worst cases, this can lead to extreme self-neglect. In addition to these problems, many present a wide range of other problems including un-intentional self-harm and harm to others, as well as possibly being vulnerable to physical, sexual, emotional and financial abuse by others. Up to about seven per cent of users experience floridly psychotic symptoms such as hallucinations and delusions, despite active pharmacological treatment. Such behaviour can result in violence, and also difficulty in cooperating and complying with medication and general care arrangements.

The age range of the users can span late adolescence to old age. The younger age group usually present the most florid and active problems and these can produce a series of family and social crises, resulting in 'revolving door' admissions to hospital on a formal basis. The older group of users additionally suffer the everyday problems of ageing and require appropriate medical interventions and care on account of their physical and sensory disabilities. Some may suffer from drug and alcohol abuse which can further complicate their mental and social functioning. A further group may begin to fall foul of the law and may require the specialised services of the forensic services.

The management of users with enduring mental illness

Pharmacotherapy

Schizophrenics will usually be given phenothiazines and other antipsychotic medication as these drugs seem to have a specific effect on the positive symptoms of schizophrenia. Those suffering from affective disorders will be given medication such as lithium or antidepressant medication which affects the mood of the individual.

Medication may be given orally but, if compliance is difficult to achieve, Depot injections may be introduced to improve cooperation; this will also allow therapeutic monitoring by the CPN at the outpatient clinic. Relapse often occurs when medication is stopped, both for those users who are taking medication therapeutically and those who take it for prevention.

Community care

Those responsible for monitoring the service user's mental health are:

* the community keyworker (CKW)
* the supervisor of the supervision register
* the supervisor of the individual's supervised discharge.

The community keyworker role has become crucial in ensuring that service users receive the appropriate care and in preventing them from falling through the care net.

It is particularly important that their specific medical and social needs are identified in the CPA and are being met and that, if changes occur, reviews are held with the appropriate members of the CPA. In addition to identifying these specific needs it is important to discover the user's more subtle and general needs. Such knowledge can usually be gained from the user, his or her carers, family and friends and other professionals involved in his or her care. Much of this understanding can only be gained in the light of experience with the user. Care plans therefore need to be sufficiently flexible to accommodate this aspect so that an overall view of the user is gained.

The complex nature of enduring mental illness requires a multidisciplinary management approach. Often the user's behaviour is fragmented, and this can lead to each professional forming a different perception of his or her needs. It can sometimes seem as if the organisations involved have taken on the user's chaotic world. It is by trying to draw together these perceptions that we can begin to get a more complete and coherent picture of the user and thereby offer the most appropriate response to his or her social, medical, human and residential needs. This process may be carried out in the CPA and the subsequent reviews of the user's care.

Expressed emotion

Social work with users with enduring mental health problems can be a delicate practice, for many fear emotional contact. Many situations which contain a high level of expressed emotion appear to produce a crisis or relapse and, for this reason, some users do better living away from their families. Social work intervention may need to be targeted on helping users and their families separate from one another and so reduce some of the harmful and intense interaction which can precipitate a crisis. Research has shown that users suffering from schizophrenia are extremely sensitive and vulnerable to their social environment (Brown *et al.*, 1958). As they tend not to be able to manage close personal relationships and social care plans CPAs should take this into account and include the provision of an appropriate environment. For example, it might be less harmful and more conducive to his or her well-being for such a user to live alone rather than to live in a situation containing a high degree of expressed emotion.

Obviously, users with enduring mental health problems share common problems but are, of course, individuals, each with their own strengths and weaknesses. Broad principles are helpful as guidelines towards creating an awareness of the particular care this group of users may require, but professionals need to be flexible to meet the individual needs of the individual user and his or her carers. For example, the social environment should not be too stimulating. It has been shown that an environment which is emotionally demanding and elicits strong feelings in the individual can soon produce further apathy and withdrawal or, alternatively, a disturbed response. The concept of expressed emotion refers to the work done with schizophrenics and their families (Leff and Vaughn, 1985). They found that not only critical comments and hostility, but also warmth and overcaring, formed what is known as high expressed emotion. The user who returns to an environment which exposes him or her to these emotions has a greater risk of relapsing to illness. Social workers should be mindful of this when making care plans and need to consider the degree of expressed emotion likely to present in a particular situation and to help friends, relatives, hostel staff, and sometimes colleagues, understand how this influences the user's behaviour.

The burden of care

We have already stressed the need for the carers and professional staff to work together with the user. Kuipers *et al.* (1989) have drawn attention to the parallels between carers and professional staff and their need to guard against burnout. The user can often make heavy demands on our resources, and these demands often seem constant and unending.

Users can often demonstrate a range of behaviour which can be very wearing and undermining to the carers and professionals involved in their care. Efforts to help can often be met by an overriding negative attitude with little or no gratitude, lack of cooperation and sabotage of care plans. In addition, users sometimes deteriorate causing their carers to feel guilty and inadequate about the help they have given. Without being supported and sharing the burden of care we can soon feel demoralised which can show itself in loss of competence, frequent absenteeism and high staff turnover. It is vital therefore that the mental health team should provide each other with a real sense of support in order to be able to contain such negative attitudes.

Until quite recently, carers' needs have not been met by other services. Despite considerable difficulties and adverse effects on their general health they have not complained much. Now carers want to become more involved with professionals in the care of users. They are no longer prepared to be passive recipients of the psychiatric services but want their contributions to be taken more seriously.

Good liaison with carers can lead to a far better understanding of users' needs and, in the long term, reduce the amount of crisis work that can occur through misunderstanding. The CPA now takes carers' needs more seriously, and their contribution towards the CPA forms a central role. Now, under the Carers Act 1995, carers have a right to have their needs assessed by the social services departments. These changes will give carers a greater and more appropriate role alongside professionals in providing care for users.

CPA care plans should be individualised to take into account the user's health and social care needs. Basic objectives should be to ensure effective provision of medication, monitor mental health and attend to physical health, nutrition, living skills, leisure, finances and accommodation. For those who are a danger to themselves or other people secure containment will need to be considered. Although we may hope for more, in terms of recovery and improvement, to maintain optimum functioning and slow down deterioration are equally valid objectives. Many of these objectives depend on being able to engage the service user, and this can sometimes be achieved with effective outreach work.

Case examples

Example 1: alleged, actual, or potential dangerousness?

The local general hospital referred a man who had recently rushed into the Casualty Department, threatened to 'shoot people', claimed he 'had a gun in his flat' but then had rushed out again. It appeared that he had later returned, and a nurse had obtained his name and address. The police would take no action, because his threat was not specific enough, and there was no evidence that he indeed had a gun.

On checking with the psychiatric unit, the approved social worker found that the man did have record of admission for mental health problems – with a past diagnosis of schizophrenia – although that was several years previously. There had been no recent contact with psychiatric services.

Given the disinclination of the police to be involved, yet with the evidence of past mental disorder, the approved social worker arranged to visit the man's GP and a psychiatrist. The GP also felt that dangerousness was not a particular issue here, which gave further cause to think that a police presence was not required.*

The assessment team convened at the patient's flat. It was a council flat with no curtains, and rather dilapidated. They knocked on the door, and the patient came to the door, wearing a flowerpot on his head. Peering over his shoulder, the team could see that the flat was almost devoid of personal possessions and rubbish was littered chaotically all over the place. The

---

* It should be noted that with more years' experience, the approved social worker, looking back on this incident, felt that this was not the way he would necessarily repeat such an assessment, taking into account the possibility that this man had earlier claimed to have a gun in his possession! We refer elsewhere in the text to issues of health and safety.

patient let them in. He agreed that he did have a gun but would not say where it was. He kept it for his own protection, because 'they' were coming after him all the time – down the chimney, through the windows, under the door, everywhere and always.

The psychiatrist said that this must be very frightening and worrying for him, and the man agreed. He said he felt that his body was infested with tiny insects, and wanted relief from these. He did not really want to go into hospital, he said, but would not put up a fight if that is what they wanted. Members of the assessment team replied, as gently as possible, that it was what they felt would be most useful for him, and might help to make him safe.

Due to the patient's ambivalence, and potential risk to others, a section for assessment was completed, although the man went amicably enough with the approved social worker and GP in the GP's car. This was a fairly unusual thing for a GP to agree to do, but there was no way in which the approved social worker could have got him to hospital alone, and it was felt by all present that the man's agreeableness was possibly temporary and needed to be capitalised upon.

Comment

It later became apparent that this man had a schizophrenic illness of a chronic and enduring kind, but which did respond positively to antipsychotic medication in that his paranoid symptoms subsided very rapidly following the commencement of medication. Given the absence of intense feelings of paranoia – and in concrete terms, this means 'fear' – this man's desperate sense of having to preserve himself also adjusted. In psychoanalytic terms, the 'gun in his flat', the threat of which precipitated the concern and therefore the assessment, might be interpreted as the gun at that moment in his own mind, which threatened him. Had an assessment not been carried out when it had been, his condition might well have deteriorated to the point where he might have felt the need to literally arm himself with a gun, to protect himself from his persecutors. The next step would then clearly have been the potential for an actual homicidal attack – possibly against the hospital, or against the next person who came to his door.

Example 2: 'burnt-out schizophrenia'?

The housing office referred a couple who were experiencing problems paying their rent. Rent would be late, not be paid in full, or the tenants would come in at odd times and appear to be quite confused. Furthermore there were reports of bullying by local children. An approved social worker visited the flat which was on the seventeenth floor of a 20-storey tower block. Windows on the communal landing were broken, and the place was cold and windy.

The approved social worker recognised the man who opened the door of the flat as someone he had known for some years in the former psychiatric hospital which had since closed. The man seemed to dimly recognise him too. He was allowed into the flat and could see that it was in a state of total chaos and disrepair. Mouldy food lay strewn around the floor, old broken records littered the chairs, and there was generally rubbish everywhere. The man had been in the flat for ten years. His last admission to hospital had been shortly before it had closed – some two years previously. He was now monitored in the community by his GP. The approved social worker discovered subsequently that he was on the waiting list for a CPN, but was not deemed of sufficiently high priority to be yet allocated one. He lived in the flat with his partner, a woman whom he had met in the psychiatric hospital and who had also been treated for many years for schizophrenia before being discharged to live independently. She was out at the time of the visit.

The man agreed that they needed some help to tidy their flat and 'keep going'; he was also worried about the local kids who taunted them. It was agreed that the approved social worker would refer them for domiciliary services, and try to help them sort out some regular arrangements for visits and contact.

When the approved social worker next visited, the man's partner was there. She too felt in need of help and advice and, after one or two more home visits, the approved social worker felt able to make an arrangement whereby they could call in and see him at the office.

Shortly after this, the woman came and began to disclose her unhappiness in their relationship and indeed how, she alleged, the male client often abused and assaulted her. With the assistance of a female co-worker, the approved social worker then began to explore this issue further, including the possibility of helping her to be rehoused.

Comment

This second example illustrates how service users can fall through the care net if they are not presenting in dramatically frightening ways, even though they might be in quite desperate need of long-term support and monitoring. Referrals can be picked up in circuitous ways – for example, through a housing problem, as in this case – yet then develop in unexpected ways – for example, the allegations of domestic violence. It might also have been helpful in this case that the approved social worker had known both clients over a very long period of time, thus enabling them to feel some sense of continuity of care, especially in the long transition to independent living.

The concept of 'burnt-out schizophrenia' tends to be a very unpopular one nowadays. It is an extremely perjorative designation if used to refer to the person rather than a description of circumstances or symptoms: in terms of sociological descriptions, we might all be said to be living in a postmodern 'burnt-out' age. 'Burnt-out schizophrenia' is an old term which was used to describe a person's state of mind where he or she had suffered from schizophrenia for many years and had grown up in the psychiatric system before the advent of effective medical treatment or community care. Such people would often have become institutionalised and emotionally stifled. Such people no longer responded to their delusional beliefs or hallucinations with the same intensity of their younger years, although would continue to experience them. Often they may have appeared unkempt, displaying peculiar or stereotyped behaviour. With the closure of the long-stay asylums and changes in attitudes, concerns have emerged that neglect and abandonment have replaced institutionalisation and abuse. The most useful way of conceptualising 'burnt-out schizophrenia' may be as follows.

People, as in the above example, who find themselves neglected by the care services – or used as political pawns in one way or another – enter a downward spiral of chaos and neglect. Workers, too, can feel themselves to be entering this downward spiral of chaos and neglect in cases where management is poor, supervision is weak or non-existent, and services are fragmented – or even sometimes at war with one another. Insofar as this creates a chaotic, persecuted and fragmentary set of services and/or organisational constraints, we might postulate the existence of the schizophrenic organisation.

Service users need to be treated with respect; therefore the designation 'burnt-out schizophrenia', insofar as it is disrespectful to the individual, must be a term of questionable usage. However, as service providers, we also need to treat each other with respect – if we do not, it seems to us that we open the doors to the creation of the schizophrenic organisation which, paradoxically, might be a helpful term, if we are to avoid its establishment!

4 Disturbances in children and adolescents

Introduction

Paediatrics is the branch of medicine which specialises in the field of childcare and childhood illnesses. Child psychiatry is specifically related to the mental and emotional difficulties which children and adolescents encounter. In addition there are other professionals interested in, and with responsibility for, childcare.

Most social workers will be acquainted with these, including GPs, schools, educational welfare departments, child guidance clinics (which are often staffed by social workers and may be headed by a consultant child psychiatrist), police, adolescent units and, of course, social work departments themselves.

The legal framework

Under the law, the person's age is taken into account when deciding on their criminal responsibility as follows:

Age	Description	Responsibility
Under 10	Child	Not criminally responsible, although may be brought to court if in need of care or control.
10–13 (inc.)	Child	Criminally responsible only if it can be proved that he or she knew that it was a wrongful act.

Age	Description	Responsibility
14–16 (inc.)	Young person	Criminally responsible.
17 and over	Adult	Criminally responsible.

Children

By 'child', in this context, we mean young people up to the time of puberty which tends to occur around the twelfth year. This is generally regarded as the time when adolescence commences.

Child development

There are many schools of thought about child development. Some of the most important seminal contributions have been theories based on psycho-sexual needs (Freud, 1905); cognitive development (Piaget, 1953), social interaction (Erikson, 1965), and learned behaviour (Skinner, 1953). Often these models devolve and become simplified to one of the most common controversies 'nature versus nurture'. In looking at development, a helpful distinction has been made by Kahn (1971) between 'biological stages' (such as naturally arise during growth) and 'cultural stages' (such as are introduced by societal patterns).

Indeed, most authorities now view human growth and development as being dependent on a number of interrelating factors, no single factor being predominant. A combination of constitutional, early experience (including, according to recent literature, pre-birth experience), parenting, social, cultural and economic factors combine to create what we know as personality. Few would argue, however, that it was Freud, through his empirical clinical work, who laid the original foundations for an understanding of childhood. For many centuries prior to this, children were perceived as little adults, rather than as new and maturing individuals. Later writers, researchers and clinicians have built on Freud's early foundations.

Childhood psychiatric difficulties tend to occur when there is either a block in development or an exaggeration of normal process. In accordance with the principle of interrelationships of factors, such difficulties can be caused in many ways, and only a full assessment, using both medical, social and psychological expertise, will reveal the causes.

For example, it is one of the tests of family therapy that an acknowledged difficulty within the family, or marital couple, will be expressed in the disturbed behaviour of either the family as a group or one member – usually a child. It is for this reason that any child with a difficulty must be assessed in the context of the family and community, rather than simply as an individual with a problem – the 'identified patient'.

Developmental milestones

The so-called 'milestones' are the stages in the child's development which mark new abilities on their path to maturity. A rough guide to these is set out in Table 4.1. As there is a wide variation in the times that different children attain these milestones, when assessing a child's maturity other factors besides physical and mental ability will need to be taken into account – factors such as their general health and well-being, their emotional state, their relationship to the outside world and, conversely, the outside world's influence on the child's immediate surroundings.

Table 4.1 Development milestones

Ability	Approximate age
Raises head; vocalises	3 months
Sits up; able to use cup	6 months
Crawls; anxious when left alone	9 months
Stands unaided; speaks first words	1 year
Picks up things from the floor; several spoken words	1–2 years
Runs; makes phrases; clean	2 years
Rides tricycle; makes sentences; sexual curiosity	3 years
Hops; speaks well	4 years
Rides bicycle; dresses and washes without help	5 years
Puberty (menarche in girls)	12 years

Childhood psychiatric disorders

Clinical syndromes have been described in attempts to classify and understand childhood difficulties.

Emotional disorders can arise in the form of fears and phobias, depression, obsessions, hysteria, shyness and elective mutism. Conduct disorders can be described as lying, fighting, and aggressive or destructive behaviour. Emotional and conduct disorders form the largest group of clinical syndromes.

Conduct disorders may only come to the notice of parents or the authorities through some kind of deviant, or persistently 'naughty' behaviour.

Certain types of behaviour are, of course, often a combination of disorders. For example, refusal to attend school is a disorder of conduct which may be accompanied by delinquent behaviour whilst away from school. It normally has, however, an emotional component in the form of a fear, phobia, or underlying depression. A further aspect of school refusal is: does the refusal lie in a fear of what is in the school or does it lie in the fear of leaving home? This question would need to be addressed in the assessment in order to ascertain the type of treatment that would be appropriate.

Psychoses

Psychoses are very rare and infrequent amongst children. Manic depression and schizophrenia rarely occur. When the symptoms of such illnesses seem to exist, they are more likely to be masking another underlying difficulty. These serious forms of psychoses do not normally have their onset until early adolescence, or later, in adult life.

Autism

Autism is the most serious psychological disorder of childhood, although it is also comparatively rare. Where it does occur, it can be observed in the earliest stages of the infant's life, and is characterised by complete withdrawal from both the parents and the world. As the child grows older, he or she will be unresponsive, lack friends and the ability to make relationships and, without treatment, will have a profound inability to speak or understand language.

Autism is more common in boys than in girls. The prognosis is not good. There remains uncertainty as to its causes, whether it is a genetic predisposition, caused by birth trauma, whether there are psychodynamic factors, or whether it is due to difficulties in the family functioning. Possible methods of treatment can therefore range from social skills training, behaviour modification or psychodynamic techniques (such as play therapy).

Hyperkinetic syndrome (ADHD)

This is a difficulty marked by excessive and continuous activity, where the child cannot stay still for very long and his or her concentration is very limited. This is more common than autism but is still comparatively rare, although recent research has indicated that it is an underdiagnosed complaint, and may occur in one child in every 200. Hyperkinetic syndrome is sometimes more commonly now referred to as ADHD (attention deficit hyperactivity disorder).

Parents, in particular, need help in acquiring the necessary skills to understand and manage their children's excited behaviour and must not be allowed to feel that they have failed because the hyperkinetic child demands knowledge and skills which parents do not normally have.

Tranquillising medication for such children is helpful in controlling some of the hyperactivity. It can also help to manage some of the more gross behaviour problems, although increasing controversy has arisen over the overprescription of such medicines as, for example, Ritalin, especially in the USA (Breggin, 1993). There is also a continuing controversy about the role of diet in treating this disorder.

Other special difficulties

There are many difficulties which may arise either briefly or for a long duration. The more common ones are: difficulties in sleeping and eating (ranging from food fads to the serious illness of anorexia nervosa); psychosomatic disorders; stammering; bedwetting (enuresis); faecal soiling (encopresis); non-accidental injuries and their effects. In addition, difficulties can arise developmentally as in cases where the child does not reach the normal milestones or perhaps surpasses them too soon. This would include such areas as slow learning, specific reading delay, general underachievement and the special problems which arise for the gifted child (who may appear bored and disinterested because he is too far ahead of his peers).

Assessments

When called to assess a child, we are faced with an immediate problem; the child has not requested us to visit. Usually either his parents or his school will have requested our assessment. In addition, we may feel that we are assessing the child in order to help him.

The child is more likely to feel that we have been called in by the authorities to chastise him or her. In such a situation we will need to consider whether the type of problem is more appropriately dealt with by an initial meeting with the child individually or together with his family.

For example, a non-accidental injury investigation may be more sensitively dealt with by a one-to-one interview; a child with a school refusal difficulty may be more appropriately seen with the family, so that any family conflicts will quickly emerge. When interviewing children it will often be helpful to do so in a quiet room, away from everyday noise. In addition, toys or plasticine should be available to give the child something to fiddle with in order to help dispel tension. In child psychotherapy such tools are invaluable, often in terms of giving the therapist information about the child's internal world. For example, dark drawings with figures of destruction will be clear clues pointing towards a child's internal turmoil and fear.

Case example

A 12 year-old boy is being referred to a special school unit on account of a learning difficulty and behaviour problems at school. He is very withdrawn and is always getting involved in fights – started by others. The social work assessment reveals that the boy is very timid – 'wet' is the word many people would apply to him – and that his mother, although very dominant and critical of the boy, is, at the same time, reluctant for him to be involved with friends of his own age. His father avoids seeing the social worker.

As the social work assessment progresses, it is revealed that the boy believes he has a worm in his tummy eating his insides. How should the social worker view the boy? Clearly, he is very miserable.

What do the symptoms mean? In an adult, the idea of a worm eating his or her insides could be seen as a delusional belief and therefore point to an incipient psychosis. This would be further indicated by the family members who would relate to each other in a way common to families with a member who becomes 'schizophrenic' – a dominant possessive mother, an absentee father and an overawed submissive male child. Alternatively, the feeling of a worm eating him may point to a potential anorexic episode (starve himself to starve the worm), although anorexia is uncommon in boys. The boy may have a fairly normal pubertal hyochondriasis; having heard somewhere that worms can live in humans, he's immediately afraid that they are in him. This would be fuelled from feelings of being attacked by external figures – the school, his mother – as if they, too, are somehow 'inside him', gnawing at his vitals.

There are no magical treatment solutions. At this stage, it is sufficient that the social worker is aware of these dimensions and can monitor the boy's progress in the special school unit for which he is being assessed. It is also important to pay close attention to the way the boy develops and whether his belief in the worm continues or alters. Through a sustained casework relationship, the social worker could do a great deal here subtly to influence the family dynamics, give the boy a greater feeling of self-worth, and help him to separate from the influence of his mother.

Methods of treatment

It is a truism to say that all children are individuals and therefore any treatment plan must take strict account of this individuality. Its practical relevance is that for any presenting difficulty – such as a tic or soiling – the assessment must attempt to understand what that particular symptom means for that particular child. There can be no such thing as dictionary of symptoms. Once such tentative understanding has been gained, there are models of treatment which can be reviewed and adopted.

The main types of treatment which are used with success are individual psychotherapy, family therapy, group psychotherapy, individual and family casework and behaviour modification. The type of treatment used must be considered alongside the venue – in particular, whether treatment is best carried out in the home or in a day, clinical or residential setting.

Medication

For dynamic, interpretative work, whether individual or family, it is preferable for the venue to be away from home – perhaps in the therapist's office, or in a quiet room without distractions. This emphasises the difference between the therapy and the home, and helps provide the patient(s) or client(s) with a container, in the form of the therapist's office and presence. If the family or individual lacks the desire to attend away from home it is unlikely that they will have the will to work towards understanding and achieve change.

Placement and, in particular, deciding whether a child should remain at home or be moved, would depend on the type of difficulty, the family and community setting. As a basic principle, the family is what the child knows, and therefore removal will inevitably tend to be disruptive. However, if his or her life or development is in severe danger – say, through repeated abuse – then removal may need to be considered.

In terms of school refusal and learning difficulties, many local authorities now have special education units, where children with these types of difficulty can be given intensive educational and casework time in order to overcome their difficulties.

Individual psychotherapy

This is carried out in a one-to-one relationship between therapist and child. The child's parent will almost certainly be seen in an initial interview, and occasionally at subsequent interviews, but the essential therapeutic process will take place in private sessions between child and therapist. The therapist will usually use play techniques, encouraging the child simply to play and describe the play.

With older children and adolescents, play can be discarded and verbal 'free association' employed (free association is the process in which the patient says whatever comes into his mind without blocking any ideas for chains of association). The therapist makes comments on this material,

interpreting from the processes that are occurring in the patient's unconscious. Thus if a child makes a plasticine mummy and daddy and the
plasticine daddy hits the plasticine mummy so she falls down, the therapist
may say something like, 'Mummies sometimes get hurt by daddies'.

Through the process of psychotherapy, the child gains a sense of internal
equilibrium and relief, and the presenting symptoms disappear. Psychotherapy is a lengthy process requiring great commitment from the therapist
and patient (or the patient's parent in bringing the child to the sessions). It
aims to resolve the underlying causes of the child's difficulties.

Family therapy

Family therapists hold the view that when a child has a presenting difficulty
this is an expression of a problem within the family structure. Thus the
family as a whole must be worked with, in an attempt to help them understand and express verbally what the problem child has been expressing with
his or her behaviour.

The advantages of family therapy over individual psychotherapy are that
it takes away the stigma and burden of the 'difficult' family member having
to carry the illness for the whole family. It is a fairly effective and economically
fast form of treatment compared to individual psychotherapy.

The disadvantages are that it relies on the commitment from the family –
who are often under other pressures from a wide variety of sources, including
social and economic ones – and relies on their ability to be able to dismiss or
present their conflicts. Often family dynamics may be so entrenched that we
can only feel grateful that we have at least one family member, albeit the
'sick' one, whom we are allowed to help. There may be a very strong vested
interest in the family maintaining the status quo.

Group psychotherapy

This is a dynamic and interpretative therapy, undertaken in a group setting.
The therapist makes interpretive comments to the group, about the group.
This can be quite a threatening experience and should be structured carefully. It is not usually applied to children but is often used for certain groups
of adolescents, mainly in clinical outpatient settings and sometimes in special
inpatient units.

Individual and family casework

This can be defined as the maintenance of a relationship with a client or
family, providing through the relationship a sense of continuity and a

facilitating environment, and playing a questioning or challenging role when that is appropriate. Social workers spend much of their time doing this; for many of their clients it seems to be a sort of a 'lifeline'.

However, it remains ill-defined, with little acknowledgement from most sources. It is hard to quantify, and harder to assess in terms of outcome, care or change. It combines a variety of theoretical positions and political possibilities and seems, in many cases, to be an appropriate method of work.

Behaviour modification

This is used frequently, often under other guises. One of the clearest examples is the use of 'positive reinforcement' in the setting of a contract between client and social worker. The client and social worker agree to perform certain acts, the mutual fulfilment of obligations resulting in, for the client, a release from his contractual duties (and for the social worker, we might add, a feeling of success).

It is also often used for specific complaints, such as enuresis. In this example, a bell and a pad could be used to ensure that, as soon as the child wets the pad on which he or she sleeps, he or she is woken by the bell. The child eventually associates wetting the bed with being woken, which leads on to him or her being able to wake before urinating, thus removing the enuretic symptom.

This works on the principle of conditioning, or deconditioning, and its proponents claim great success in many areas, such as enuresis, fears and phobias and certain types of antisocial behaviour. Behaviour modification aims to remove the symptoms of a particular form of difficult or distressing behaviour. It does not attempt to deal in any way with its underlying causes.

Children of mentally ill parents

This is a client group for whom social workers can play a very helpful and important role, both in terms of ongoing support over a period of years and also in times of crisis during hospital admissions. Children of mentally ill parents are in a vulnerable and sensitive position and are at much greater risk than children in families where there is no history of, nor any current, mental illness (Rutter, 1974, 1981; Woodley, 1995).

The types of risk vary, according to whether the mental illness has been an ongoing difficulty for the parent – say, in the case of manic depressive illness or neurotic disorders which require long-term therapeutic support – or whether the mental illness is clearly of short-term duration – say, in the case of puerperal psychosis precipitated by childbirth.

Long-term mental illness

In the case of a long-term mental illness, children will clearly need casework help in the form of an opportunity to explore and accept their parent's illness and its vicissitudes (its unpredictability, its confusion and its misery). This will take many hours of patient counselling.

Some children may not be able to speak about their feelings. Others will give the impression that they have no problems whatsoever. This can be a more worrying indication because it probably means that the child is denying any problems and that his or her worries have gone underground and may resurface later. Hudson (1982) has highlighted the worrying implications of 'modelling', where the child models his behaviour on his parents who in turn may well be behaving quite bizarrely. Unless there is a risk of physical danger, it is generally preferable to support such a family with the children staying at home. Social workers will be guided on this by the wishes of the children and the level of home care the parent(s) are able to provide.

Short-term mental illness

In the case of short-term illness or crisis – in particular puerperal psychosis which is a severe psychotic episode of a time-limited duration – there is less necessity for long-term casework but a reliance must be placed on the statutory services, including the social worker, to take control and manage the situation. It is at times of crisis that the issue of whether to remove the child or not becomes of prime importance.

The psychotic parent may have a delusional belief about the child or infant – for example, that their baby is a time bomb waiting to explode. In this situation the child may be at great risk. Removal from the mother could be indicated if the child were, say, two or three years old. Where the child is a newborn baby, then both mother and baby could be admitted together into a special hospital unit, to allow bonding to continue, but in a supported and monitored setting.

The well parent

The other parent – the 'well' parent – can often be relied on to manage the situation and ensure that he or she is compensated for any severe deprivation. However, the social worker must be sensitive to this parent's needs also, and support can be given to them. 'Support' can often be something as basic as an occasional telephone call, although it can be more. For example, the social worker can supervise meetings between the violent psychotic parent and his wife and children thereby ensuring that no harm comes to the wife and children, while still giving them the opportunity to keep in touch with the father.

Preventive measures

When a child has mentally ill parents, preventive measures can be employed to try to ensure that any future emotional difficulties are minimised. For example, where the mother suffers from an enduring mental illness and there is evidence that she had this illness when her child was born, then it may be appropriate for the social worker to discuss with the mother referring the child to a child guidance clinic for outpatient psychotherapy. This can commence as early as the child's third year and can help bring out and resolve any underlying unconscious difficulties. In addition, more immediately practical resources can be offered, such as nurseries, childminding, playgroups, mother and baby groups and other self-help groups. In these ways, the child's mother may be given support by her peers without depriving her of her role as mother.

Unless resolved at an early stage, such difficulties may lie submerged until the time of puberty, which tends to act as a trigger for the replay of very early infant difficulties. This is one reason why many adult psychotic illnesses are precipitated around the time of adolescence.

Adolescents

We have seen that the child experiences rapid physical growth until the later years of childhood when the pace slows down and early conflicts are put aside for a time. This is the calm before the storm. Adolescence is then marked by physical changes with the onset of puberty; this, together with psychological, academic and other pressures, combine to produce considerable stress.

The young person's degree of disturbance and his or her ability to cope with it will be largely determined by the quality of care he has received as a child, and is now receiving, from his parents. For it is in adolescence that early childhood experiences and difficulties reawaken, to come to the fore again. All these rapid changes call for great powers of readjustment which inevitably lead, in many cases, either to emotional disturbance experienced internally as feeling or acted out externally in behaviour. Most adolescents survive these stresses (as do their parents). Any interference in the individual's capacity to cope is usually temporary and related to some developmental stress already mentioned.

The young person may become depressed, feel anxious and have doubts about him or herself, but these pass and give rise to firmer plans about the future. Invariably this period is marked by alternating attitudes of wanting to become independent whilst at the same time seeking the care and support of parents. This is, therefore, generally a time of stress for parents too.

Identity crisis

The central task of the adolescent is to establish the issue of his or her own identity. Before this time of transition, his or her identity will largely have been determined for him or her by his or her family, school and peer group. He or she will now be faced with shaping a role for him or herself, which often means a struggle towards independence, away from the security afforded by parents and friends, from home to community. The adolescent will be seeking a place for him or herself in the adult world.

The crisis of identity is a particularly useful concept for those concerned with helping adolescents. It can give focus and goal towards guiding them through their diffused and distressed (and distressing) behaviour, and into more mature relationships with their world. The behaviour problems expressed by young people in their quest for identity may range from acts of destructiveness against family and property to complaints that he or she is unable to make friendships to failing to fulfil academic potential at school. There may be experiences of emptiness, depression or isolation.

Neurotic and psychotic disorders

We can now perhaps see how the normal stresses of adolescence can trigger off more profound problems which may have lain dormant since early childhood. These are usually related to failure in one of the developmental tasks – a failure which, if not corrected by skilled help, may begin to restrict the young person's emotional growth, and make attachments difficult.

It is in this area that skilled psychotherapy is indicated. Often these problems make it difficult for the young person to change their relationships with their parents and they may reach adulthood with no close relationships. The adolescent may find it difficult to come to terms with their bodies, and in particular with their dawning sexual feelings. They may feel that their bodies are not their own, that they are still the property of their parents, giving rise to guilt and disorientation.

Neurotic disturbances

Neurotic disturbance in adolescence has been differentiated by Laufer

(1975) into two subdivisions: 'simple neurotic disturbance' in which the internal conflict does not appear to seriously interfere with the young person's life but does reduce the level of his functioning; and 'serious neurotic disturbance' in which there is a more longstanding deadlock within the individual, interrupting his or her functioning. In both types of disturbance, the adolescent does not lose contact with external reality and is able to draw distinctions between the reactions of the external world and his or her own mind.

When assessing the extent of adolescent disturbance it is important to bear in mind the age of the young person and the 'age appropriateness' of his behaviour. For example, a boy of 13 who is awkward and feels unable to allow himself to masturbate may be expressing temporary stress without it being a sign of permanent disorder.

If the boy is still unable to masturbate at 18, this may be expressing a fear of his own sexual feelings. A similar example could be the instance of a girl of 13 who is unable to go to a party because she is shy with boys and feels herself to be unattractive. In this instance, she may be showing signs of age-related stress. However, if the same girl is 18 and is still unable to go to parties, she may be demonstrating an inability to allow herself to be a grown-up woman; this, at the age of 18, would indicate an established disturbance with which she would need help.

Psychotic disorders

The more severe forms of mental illness can occur in adolescence. It is critical to be able to distinguish between them and normal adolescent problems. It must be emphasised that while the personality is still not fully formed, psychiatric diagnosis is notoriously difficult and unreliable, let alone indicative of prognosis and outcome. Made too definitively, it can lead to a premature and inappropriate labelling of the person.

Broadly speaking, we should regard the adolescent as mentally ill if he or she has lost touch with reality. A psychotic disorder is usually more permanent and fixed than the transitory neurotic disturbance. The young person's thought, memory and movement are all affected and he or she will seem convinced that what his or her mind is creating – his or her 'internal world' – is true and real, irrespective of what is occurring in his or her home, school, work and social surroundings – his or her 'external world'.

Many people think that mental illness is obvious and that it requires little skill to be able to tell the difference between 'madness' and disturbed behaviour. Nothing could be further from the truth. The psychotic process can be quiet and slow in progression; it requires the expertise of a skilled psychiatrist to be able to make a sound diagnosis.

Schizophrenia and manic depressive illnesses

Schizophrenia and manic depressive illness often have their onset in adolescence. It is therefore imperative to refer the adolescent for help where there are any indications that his or her behaviour suggests such a mental disorder.

Other disturbances

Among the emotional disturbances that may occur and need to be referred for treatment are sexual problems (for example, promiscuity or concern and confusion about sexual identity), deliberate self-harm, obesity, solvent abuse, problem drinking or drug-taking. Some of these issues ar dealt with in more detail in Chapter 8.

Behaviour – particularly delinquent behaviour, such as burglary, stealing cars, compulsive lying, gambling, repeated drunkenness or theft – can also be indicative of underlying emotional conflicts.

Where such behaviour is evident and persistent, a full assessment is indicated in order to understand and, where appropriate, treat a person's difficulties.

Treatment

Most adolescents come through their difficult passage and reach adulthood. Some, however, will need help to achieve this. In the case of the neurotic and psychotic individuals, psychiatric treatment will be essential to prevent the illness from deteriorating and blocking further development towards maturity.

Most young people who need psychiatric help can be treated as outpatients with a combination of individual and group psychotherapy, and occasionally medication. More severe instances may require inpatient treatment in special adolescent units where, parallel with treatment, the young person may have special tuition so that he or she is not left behind academically.

The sociological perspective

In addition to the pressures created for adolescents by their own feelings, there is, of course, the difficulties which come, or seem to come, from others around him. These difficulties can, by their nature, seem incomprehensible to those closest to the young person. They can include such factors as the pressure from the parents to 'grow up', 'sort yourself out' or 'conform' or pressure from society to work, study and succeed. Such pressures may seem to be of doubtful value at a time of economic and cultural uncertainty.

One response to these pressures can be to become mentally ill. Another is to align with an alternative culture: the attraction of gangs, ideological movements and youth sub-elites, has been well documented, especially since the early 1960s. One could list such examples as 'teddy boys', 'rockers', 'mods', 'hell's angels', 'hippies', 'skinheads', 'rastas' and 'punks' (Leech, 1975; Hall and Jefferson, 1975).

This is clearly an area where psychological and sociological understanding would need to merge in the assessment process. For instance, a 14 year-old punk girl who sniffs glue may be telling us more about the cultural norms of the subgroup to which she has chosen to belong than she is about her own individual psychopathology.

5 Mental impairment, learning disability and difficulty

Introduction

In the chapter entitled 'Euphemisms and abuse' in her book, *Mental Handicap and the Human Condition* (1994), Valerie Sinason offers some 43 differing descriptions, ranging from the sixteenth century to the present day, which have been used at various times to describe what we now refer to variously as learning disability, learning difficulty, mental handicap, or in the terms of the Mental Health Act 1983, 'mental impairment, or severe mental impairment'. Learning disability tends to be the preferred term for common usage and is used in the World Health Organisation definitions, although this term actually dates back to 1492 when it meant 'want of ability, impotence leading to legal disqualification ... It denotes a restriction resulting from an organic impairment' (Sinason, 1994, p.44). Sinason goes on to state that 'impaired' means 'unequal; unsuitable (1606); odd, made worse (1839)' (ibid., p.45), although this term, again, has been revived to be used in the WHO definition of handicap, as well as in the Mental Health Act 1983, as we shall go on to discuss. The usage of words seems to have been especially important in relation to learning disability because of the immense abuse which has been inherent in the terminology used, implying that the person and the disability are one and the same and that he or she is a disabled person, rather than someone experiencing a disability of some kind.

To turn this viewpoint around, the recent focus on normalisation, or disabling society, has shown that it is society's reactions – indeed, our own reactions and perceptions – which creates the disabled atmosphere in which people are not permitted or encouraged to be able. Such a perspective might be illustrated in the very definition of learning disability which involves IQ ratings, so that the person's score on the IQ scale formed his or her own personal definition. Hence, IQ ranges of 50–70 indicated a mild or moderate handicap, an IQ below 50 indicated a severe handicap, whilst below 24 indicated a profound handicap. Quite how IQ ratings are measured, and what they mean, however, might be subject to question. As Sinason observes such scores are 'just one useful indicator of cognitive functioning' (ibid., p.10).

In her book Sinason goes on to illustrate some of her work in the field of psychotherapy with people who have experienced a learning disability. Axiline (1976) has illustrated the long-term psychotherapy of a child with a diagnosis of autism. The UCH *Textbook of Psychiatry* (Wolff *et al.*, 1991) describes the broad range of types of difficulties included under the broad heading 'mental impairment' and, before going on to consider how these might become manifested such that a referral under the Mental Health Act is made necessary, it is perhaps worthwhile pausing to clarify what some of the main categories are.

Moving away from the consideration of descriptive terms, and the tendency towards value differentiation as a result of terminology, a learning disability is generally ascribed when there is an observable difficulty in mental functioning as a result of an organic cause. Some such difficulties can arise as a consequence of genetic factors, (Hurler's syndrome, Hunter's syndrome, tuberous sclerosis), chromosomal factors (Down's syndrome, cri du chat syndrome, Fragile X syndrome, prenatal complications (rubella, toxoplasmosis), perinatal complications (prematurity, anoxia, birth trauma), or postnatal developments (epilepsy, infections, lead poisoning).

Autism is a disorder characterised by withdrawal from contact, an inability to develop language and, occasionally, ritualised behaviour. It can also be accompanied by extraordinary gifted powers in a particular area, the cinematic portrayal of *The Rain Man* being a recent and rather classic example of a case of autism extending into adult life, where such a later diagnosis might become one of Asperger's Syndrome (Wing, 1981; Rutter, 1985).

Turning now to the Mental Health Act 1983 we find the definition, for its purposes, of 'severe mental impairment' as being a condition where there is 'arrested or incomplete development of mind which includes severe impairment of intelligence and social functioning and is associated with abnormally aggressive or seriously irresponsible conduct on the part of the person concerned' (section 1 (2)), while 'mental impairment' means arrested or incomplete development of mind (not amounting to severe mental impairment) which includes significant impairment of intelligence and social functioning and is associated with abnormally aggressive or seriously irresponsible conduct on the part of the person concerned' (ibid.).

Taking into account the controversy around the use and abuse of terminology as in 'arrested or incomplete development of mind ...' and so on, the key for the approved aocial worker, in relation to assessment of risk, appears to lie in the judgement of what constitutes 'abnormally aggressive or seriously irresponsible conduct ...' in the life of the individual concerned and those immediately close to that person.

Chapter 29 of the Mental Health Act Commission Code of Practice attempts to offer some guidance on this. As observed there, it is true to say that very few people with a learning difficulty are detained under the Mental Health Act.

Where a referral arises for a person with a learning disability, or where it emerges during the course of the assessment that a person has a learning disability, then reference must immediately be made to a consultant psychiatrist and/or social worker with specialist knowledge in this area. In the absence of such a specialist, detention under section 4 or 2 for an assessment, is likely to be preferable, rather than detention under section 3 for treatment. Given the difficulties which can arise in communication, these factors are also important in situations where a social worker is involved in intervention under the Police and Criminal Evidence Act 1984 – given the propensity for people with a learning disability to confess to crimes which they have not committed – as well as for advice and consultation in cases of referral for guardianship, bearing in mind the loss of life in the Beverley Lewis case (Fennell, 1989).

Case examples

Example 1: independent living

A referral to the mental health crisis team was made by a consultant psychiatrist specialising in learning disability. The subject of the referral was a young man who had been placed in a group living situation in a tower block some years previously. One by one, the three other residents had moved out into their own flats, leaving this young man living alone in a four-bedroomed flat, several floors up. He had a learning disability but had been diagnosed in the past as experiencing psychotic episodes.

Once upon a time, support tenants had lived in a flat next door to this young man's four-bedroomed tenancy, but they too had moved on, and their flat had been let to tenants not involved in any support scheme – they just lived there as council tenants, minding their own business.

This referral came about because the young man had been the subject of numerous case conferences over the previous few years, each case conference identifying support needs, but with less support subsequently materialising. The consultant was therefore concerned generally about the way in which social and health services were neglecting this young man in the context of his learning disability, his increasing loneliness and isolation, as well as by the new development of reports from neighbours – not only from those in the erstwhile support tenancy, but from others too – of hearing screams, banging, and drilling emanating from the flat. During previous paranoid episodes, this young man had injured himself, and had come to the attention of police for presenting frightening and threatening behaviour to others.

An assessment was arranged, and on the strong advice, recommendation and encouragement from the consultant who had known this young man for many years, a substantial police presence was requested in order to restrain the client from harming others or himself.

A section 135 warrant was obtained, again, following advice that the consultant and members of his team had attempted to visit and engage the young man in informal intervention, but access had been refused and in-coherent abuse had been hurled at them through the – apparently barricaded – door.

On arrival at the flat, the approved social worker saw that the door was indeed barricaded. The polite request for the door to be opened, with the explanation as to why, was greeted from within by loud moans and screams. The assessment team then heard doors banging and, suddenly, the sound of loud drilling. The police, at the sounds from within, summoned back-up, and a number of officers arrived with plastic shields and body armour. The door was forced, and access was gained; following a swift search of the flat, the young man was found and overpowered with diffi-culty, given the presence of sharp instruments, including a hand drill. Looking around the bare walls, the approved social worker saw that the young man had been engaged in drilling holes and pulling away great chunks of plaster, as well as smearing the walls with food and other sub-stances – possibly excrement.

The approved social worker and consultant tried to speak to the young man, to try to attempt an interview in an appropriate manner, but he seemed quite disorientated, shouted incoherently and could give no explanation of who he was, what was on his mind, or why he appeared to be ripping apart the flat.

Indeed, so distressing were the circumstances of this assessment that the police themselves appeared upset at having to restrain someone who was unwell. The young man was admitted to hospital under section 3 and, over the next few months, recovered and was later rehoused into more supportive accommodation.

Comment

This example highlights again the way in which the cycle of neglect seems to perpetuate an abusive system. It is relatively easy for services to discover bureaucratic impediments to allocating cases, or time or space over periods of weeks, months or years. In the matter of learning disability and mental health, however – the area of 'dual disability' – such distancing of services leads to a multiplication of risk factors in the long term. In this example, at the end of the process of neglect, the young man was displaying seriously irresponsible and potentially aggressive behaviour. Nevertheless, these circumstances were probably preventable. Working together with a professional who knew the client and who was an expert in the field helped contain the worst risk factors, although the indignity which the client was forced to experience was not beneficial, and any paranoid feelings which he might have already been experiencing were certainly given cause and foundation by the end of that particular assessment.

Example 2: anxiety and learning disability

A concerned day centre worker referred their mentally ill client for assessment because she was young (although over 18) and 'open to exploitation'. She had previously been homeless but had moved into a young man's flat, and he had 'learning difficulties'. The day centre worker had a real cause for anxiety generally about the female client, because she had been homeless, had a history of admissions to psychiatric hospitals and might therefore be at some risk – returning from another direction, to the Beverley Lewis dilemmas, perhaps. For these reasons, an approved social worker and colleague did attempt to visit the young woman at the address given. She was not at home, but the tenant was. The tenant had no difficulty in discussing with the approved social worker his relationship with the young woman and the fact that she stayed there sometimes, but they were friends and tried to take care of each other. This seemed perfectly reasonable and human, with few elements of risk attached – and certainly no significantly greater risks than in many other relationships. Therefore no further action was taken in this case to try to force any intervention or assessment.

Comment

This example highlights how an approved social worker needs to enter each situation with an open mind. Whilst recognising the many levels of potential and actual risk there is also the need to retain one's humanity and sensitivity to individuals' situations and circumstances.

It also raises the issue of sexuality and people's right to choose and express their sexuality – something which people with learning disabilities have had to struggle for, against prejudice.

6 Older people

Introduction

About two-thirds of referrals to social services departments concern older people. Although these referrals may often be for practical services such as home care or meals on wheels, they can often conceal considerable unmet needs. Research has shown that many older people who suffer from dementia and depression do not receive the help they require because they have not been diagnosed or identified as needing treatment.

With the growing number of older people in the population this has become a matter of increasing concern. Depression and dementia are the two main mental health problems that affect older people. Over 6 per cent of those over 65 suffer from dementia and about 15 per cent suffer from depression which would warrant treatment. The rate is higher in those aged over 80.

Before we begin to consider some of the mental health problems that affect older people, we should remind ourselves that old age itself is not a condition but a stage of life, and that people bring to it their own unique life experiences and personalities. One common factor that older people share to differing degrees is a sense of depletion and this usually takes the form of diminished sight, hearing and mobility as well as, often, reduced living standards due to reduced financial circumstances. Old age can be a time of increased dependency and vulnerability and this can make it difficult for some older people to manage their own lives.

All these problems can be compounded if the family has dispersed and the spouse has died, leaving the old person isolated and without support. Many older people's mental health problems have special features and, for this reason, we have decided to present them separately in this chapter.

Bereavement

Older people are subject to bereavement of family and friends. These experiences can reawaken earlier losses and, if these were not dealt with adequately at the time, they can play a significant role in producing depression and can serve to further undermine the person's mental health. The final phase of life could be said to be characterized by mourning – mourning retirement, loss of contact with colleagues and creative work and mourning of life itself.

Perhaps the loss of a life partner is the most painful loss of all. Although both partners may live with the knowledge that the cost of their commitment to each other means eventual separation through death, when one partner dies the one that is left behind may feel lost and doubt their ability to cope alone. At times of crises older people need the support of family, and sometimes professionals, to help them through their grief. Some bereavement services tend to concentrate on those users who have lost someone through illness or accident. Yet older people can often suffer from multiple bereavements of family and friends, leaving them isolated and more vulnerable.

Most older people have the strength and character to cope with such losses, others will not, and may need the care of others to enable them to work through their sadness and loss. Without such help, many may continue to be depressed and neglect their diet and care leaving them more prone to physical illness, social isolation and, sometimes, suicide.

Feeling depressed can sometimes make people inarticulate and isolated; they can feel unworthy of others' interest and concern and therefore may not ask for help. Primary medical and psychiatric services need to be sensitive to these issues, for much of the depression suffered by older people may be hidden or expressed in psychological and physical guises such as confusion, vague aches and pains – in fact, many of the ailments that older people complain about.

Affective disorders

The most common affective disorder in old age is depression which may be related to some of the stresses already mentioned. Depression can present as extreme sadness or, more subtly, it can manifest as self-neglect and in many confusional guises. In addition, it can take the form of vague aches and pains and preoccupation with the state of health.

Confusional behaviour resulting from depression can sometimes be misdiagnosed as dementia.

Depression varies in degree from feelings of sadness and a sense of loneliness to the most profound clinical depression sometimes referred to as endogenous depression. The main characteristics of this kind of illness are loss of drive, appetite, poor sleep and difficulty in concentration. The person will often feel worse in the morning when he or she will waken early but may then feel better as the day proceeds. Preoccupation with bowel symptoms, including constipation and hypochrondriacal fears of cancer and other ailments are not uncommon. Severe retardation can produce mutism; difficulty in thinking and making decisions can often make the person totally inaccessible.

Hypomania

Hypomania can be the reverse of depression. It is a rarer condition and occurs in about 5 per cent of affective disorders in older people. The hypomanic episode usually alternates between bouts of depression. In between these episodes of mania and depression there can be long periods of normality.

In the hypomanic phase the person is usually bursting with ideas and energy with pressures of speech. He or she can be reckless, spending money on items which he or she cannot afford or does not need. Such behaviour can soon lead to debts and, if intervention does not take place, financial ruin. He or she may also show great irritability; indeed, this may be the first sign of the illness. If he or she is obstructed or feels thwarted he or she may react with aggression.

Many manic patients do not sleep or eat well, and this can soon present considerable risk to their general health. Another special feature which is present at the outset in older manic patients is confusion which can lead to a misdiagnosis of delirium. Paranoid ideas may be expressed and they may become frankly deluded and experience hallucinations.

Whilst in this state of mind it is difficult for their families or professionals to gain their cooperation. Although hypomania is less severe in older people than in other age groups, it requires prompt intervention with medication to get it under control, usually on an inpatient basis.

Senile dementia

The most common and most serious demential illness is called Alzheimer type (SDAT). In its rarer form, when it occurs before the age of, say, 65, it is referred to as pre-senile dementia and, after this age, senile dementia. It seems to be found predominantly in women. In the pre-senile type of dementia, there is a more rapid decline, the main characteristics being a decline in intellect, personality and behaviour. The most marked early symptoms are emotional disturbance, paranoid ideas, personality change, plus forgetfulness with loss of recent memory. The latter symptoms are due to the fact that the person is no longer able to learn new information.

Disorientation and an inability to think conceptually are prominent features. Memory of the remote past may remain intact, and this may account for so many patients with this disorder dwelling in the past. In the early stages the patients may have insight into their condition and their change in behaviour and memory loss, which may lead to understandable pain and distress to both the patients and their families.

As the condition insidiously progresses, there is increased deterioration in social functioning to the point where patients are unable to perform simple daily tasks, such as dressing and feeding. This can soon lead to personal neglect and carelessness. Disorientation may then occur first in time, then in place and person, until they are unable to recognise their nearest and dearest.

This makes it extremely difficult for carers to look after such patients. They will require considerable help and support in both practical and emotional terms, if the care is not to break down. It is often the behaviour problems which include wandering, asking the same question over and over again, the odd sleep patterns and aggressive outbursts that lead to distress and exhaustion in their carers.

Acute confusional states

Delirium states are common in older people and can lead to very disturbed behaviour. These may be the result of a number of stresses which are usually physical but sometimes psychological. Physical stresses are usually caused by acute infections such as pneumonia, and these can soon be brought under control by the administration of antibiotics, often before the more florid states develop.

Although such conditions are usually treated in general hospitals, these patients may be encountered by approved social workers because of the disturbed behaviour associated with such conditions. The onset from normality to acute disturbance can occur within a few days.

Confusion is often a prominent symptom, and this is more marked in the evenings and at night when the light fails and the patient is unable to perceive his or her familiar surroundings. The patient then becomes disorientated and bewildered, and as a result, can often experience terrifying visual hallucinations. Disorientation is increased if the patient is transferred to an unfamiliar place. Memory of recent events may be lost and the patient may make paranoid interpretations of events around him or her. His or her thinking is often disjointed and speech may either be slow or, alternatively, accelerated. He or she also suffers from clouding of consciousness and limited concentration, becoming restless and failing to grasp and maintain basic information. He or she may begin to roam round the house or take to wandering the streets, searching in his or her delirium.

Common causes of delirium states

- infections affecting the lungs, such as bronchitis or pneumonia, and urinary infections which are common in the elderly
- malnutrition
- dehydration
- metabolic and endocrine disorders – for example, diabetes, intoxication of drugs and alcohol, trauma of the head, hypothermia.

Multi-infarct (arthroscleratic) dementia

This type of dementia is the result of a deprived blood supply to the brain which is usually caused by a series of minor strokes, and hardening and thickening of the arteries. Because parts of the brain are cut off from a blood supply, the brain cells die and cannot replace themselves, causing permanent damage. This disorder is often associated with high blood pressure and seems to affect more men than women. The average age of onset is around 60.

Unlike senile dementia there is often a sudden onset which produces episodes of confusion, slurring of speech and weakness down one side of the body. Sometimes the blood circulation is restored to the affected part of the brain which leads to some improvement and, in some cases, full recovery. However, most cases suffer a subsequent episode within a matter of weeks or months. After a succession of such episodes, recovery is often less marked, and the process leads to the characteristic 'step ladder' deterioration of personality with obvious dementia.

Confusion in this type of dementia differs from that found in other dementias. For example, patients may be very muddled in the morning and become lucid and alert in the afternoon, only to return to wandering and disorientation in the evening. Patients are often very emotional and this may well be related to the fact that their personalities are still well preserved until the late stage of the illness.

Patients retain insight into their condition of failing memory and this can cause them profound depression and, in some cases, to commit suicide.

As in other dementias, paranoid phases may be present. Patients will be sensitive to their memory deficit. This can be seen as an understandable defence manoeuvre. Paranoid attitudes do not have the same elaborate system found in paraphrenia (see below) or other paranoid conditions of old age.

Paranoid attitudes, where present, are often directed towards those people close at hand, especially relatives or those caring for the person.

Schizophrenia and paraphrenia

Schizophrenia in older people can be the result of lifelong illness which has persisted into old age. Such people may continue to suffer from the severe residual defects of the disorder – blunted emotions, delusions and auditory hallucinations. Schizophrenia can also occur for the first time in old age, and this condition is known as paraphrenia.

Such disorders are usually predominantly found in women who live solitary lifestyles and who are often partially deaf. Although they may have always been regarded as somewhat eccentric they usually have no history of serious psychiatric illness.

The illness often occurs over the age of 65 and those presenting problems are invariably very bizarre with paranoid delusions relating to their neighbours. They are unlike younger paranoid patients in the sense that the suspicions are localised to the people living upstairs or next door, and do not usually involve people in their wider world. Such paranoid delusions seldom alter but are held and sustained with strong intensity. They are also systematised and contain the most extraordinary sexual ideas and a sense of terrifying persecution.

Because of the troublesome effects of such a disorder it is unlikely to go unnoticed, for the people affected are likely to complain loudly about their imaginary persecutors. They are most commonly referred to the social services as a result of a request for rehousing but this is not likely to be very successful in the majority of cases, for such patients take their delusional system with them and soon begin to complain again with the same delusional ideas.

Like delusions in other disorders it is fruitless to argue with people thus affected. It is important to acknowledge how frightened such experiences must make them feel and convey this to them without colluding with their delusions.

Treatment

Because it is often difficult to gain the trust of such suspicious individuals it is important to enlist the help of the community psychiatric nurse and the patient's GP. Medication along the lines given to paranoid schizophrenics is often helpful in diminishing the intense persecution of the delusions and hallucinations that such people suffer. Intramuscular injections of either

Modecate or Depixol can be given at prescribed intervals which can range from one to several weeks.

If the patient is acutely disturbed it may be necessary to admit him or her to hospital for assessment and treatment. Such patients often welcome this to give them some respite from their persecutors, but if an assessment can be made as an outpatient this can be sufficient.

Insight is rarely obtained and it is usually necessary for the paraphrenic to remain under psychiatric supervision for the rest of their life. Day care can be a very helpful resource, once the trust of the elderly person has been gained.

Mental health in elders: case examples

Example 1: feeding pigeons

A 61 year-old lady was referred to the social services by housing department officials and neighbours. The whole local community felt that she was risking her health and that of others because she fed pigeons on her balcony in such large numbers that flocks of birds would descend perpetually.

Under some pressure from her seniors, the approved social worker visited the lady. She was not in, but there was a stomach-churning smell emanating from inside her flat. The approved social worker returned very early one morning, with the lady's GP (who, incidentally, had not seen her for years). The lady was in, and opened the door a crack. The smell was really dreadful as the door was opened. The lady was dirty and dishevelled. She would not let them in she said, because she could not open the door. It was jammed. She wanted no help. She was OK. She slammed the door in their faces. The approved social worker felt that she had sufficient ground to request a section 135 warrant in order to obtain access to assess the lady's mental health.

It must be remembered that a section 135 does not require the approved social worker to know that a person requires admission – merely that they have 'reasonable cause to suspect that' assessment for admission is necessary. The section 135 was obtained and, early one morning, the approved social worker returned, together with the GP, a psychiatrist and a policeman.* The lady was in her flat, but adamantly refused to let anyone in, or open the door.

---

* Section 135 empowers a police constable to force access, accompanied by an approved social worker and a GP; properly speaking it is not the approved social worker who ought to be forcing access, although the section 135 must be requested by an approved social worker.

On forcing access, the approved social worker found the flat to be packed with rubbish in carrier bags of all descriptions, shapes and sizes. Indeed, it was quite hard to open the door, such was the volume of rubbish. The lady could give no coherent account of how she was living, or why she was choosing to live as she was; but in view of the health hazard, and her apparent malnutrition, the assessment team felt that a section 2 assessment was justified. She was admitted to hospital, but no psychotic symptoms emerged except for a degree of vagueness, such as to suggest possible simple schizophrenia. Consequently, the lady was discharged at the end of her 28 days and immediately resumed her lifestyle of collecting rubbish from the streets and bringing it home, interspersed with periods of feeding the pigeons.

Comment

It might be asked, 'What was the point of this assessment?' Does it indicate that the approved social worker was wrong and overstepped her authority? The problem here was that, outwardly, the lady was placing her health at risk by attracting hordes of pigeons but was also collecting smelly rubbish and not taking sufficient care of herself – not eating nourishing food and so on. There were therefore probably sufficient indications that, had a section 2 not been initiated after an assessment, the approved social worker could have been held liable should anything subsequently have happened to this lady. The case therefore involved an element of defensive practice. Furthermore, the lady was in danger of losing her tenancy as a nuisance, and becoming intentionally homeless. Therefore, it was, arguably, correct to ensure that she was given every opportunity to receive proper and adequate treatment – notwithstanding the fact that she did not want this.

Example 2: husband and wife

A 70 year-old man had suffered a manic depressive illness over some years, controlled through medication, but with occasional periods requiring inpatient treatment. He seemed to be becoming depressed, and his wife asked the social services for help. Due to staff shortages, an assessment was rather slow in taking place.

One day, the man went missing, and his wife desperately pleaded with the social services to be available to help when he returned. He was found by the police and not knowing his history, but finding his address in his wallet, they returned him to his home.

Later that day, he assaulted his wife. An approved social worker visited but, by then, found that the man had become mute and virtually catatonic.

Together with the GP and a psychiatrist, the approved social worker completed an assessment and placed him under section 3. He had to be lifted bodily into the ambulance, with the assistance of police, because by that point he had allowed his body to become limp and totally refused to cooperate.

Comment

This example illustrates that it is important for approved social workers and other professionals to take seriously the concerns of relatives. When unwell, people can become a great risk to themselves or others, reacting in ways which appear unpredictable to those who do not know them. However for those close to them, such patterns can be predicted.

In listening to the testimony of relatives, there must always be an element of caution, if not scepticism, in case any relationship problems or disputes are clouding the issue or affecting the description of a person's behaviour. However, taking that reservation into account, carers are entitled to be accorded credibility and in cases of severe mental illness – where a person's delusions might lead them to confabulate, for example – the relative may well be the only, and most reliable, witness who will ultimately make the difference between life and death of the person being assessed.

7 Culture and diversity

Introduction

In this chapter we consider briefly some of the contemporary debates and theoretical positions around culture and diversity. As these are such complex debates, we do not propose to be able to cover every perspective. Rather, our discussion will focus on the approved social worker's role in exemplifying good practice under the Mental Health Act 1983. In this way, our approach is admittedly modest yet, in so being, is based on an acceptance of diversity and preparedness to be open to newness and development.

The legislative imperative to pay respect to the individuality and 'difference' of the other person lies in section 13 (2) of the Mental Health Act, where it is stated that:

> Before making an application for admission of a patient to hospital an Approved Social Worker shall interview the patient in a suitable manner and satisfy himself that detention in a hospital is in all manner of the circumstances of the case the most appropriate way of providing the care and medical treatment of which the patient stands in need. (Mental Health Act 1983, quoted in Jones, 1996: 70)

In his commentary on the above paragraph, Jones states:

> The words 'suitable manner' should direct the Approved Social Worker's attention to the needs of all groups, including children, who might have difficulty communicating effectively. (Jones, 1996: 73)

This could include people who are deaf, as well as people whose first language is not English, but might also include people who are born in this country but whose mother tongue is not English and who may be using an alternative language to English as a result of distress to which they feel subject. Before making a judgement therefore about the possible need or otherwise for hospital admission or treatment under compulsion, the approved social worker must do all he or she can to ensure that the person being assessed has had the best possible opportunity to be understood by the assessment team.

Being understood, however, clearly does not relate to language alone. Cultural factors also come into play, and approved social workers need to do what they can to become conversant with the cultural values and religious beliefs of the communities they serve in order to be prepared to be culturally sensitive during assessments. Clearly, no one can know or retain every fact about every culture – especially approved social workers in airports, inner-city casualty units or major railway termini – so, as well as knowledge, they also need a flexibility of approach, an open mind, and a value-free attitude when it comes to intervening and assessing the lives, actions and beliefs of others. These factors are increasingly relevant in today's postmodern society in which international travel and migration patterns have become increasingly flexible and possible.

With particular reference to what the Mental Health Act Commission in their *Sixth Biennial Report 1993–5* term 'Ethnic issues', such issues have been particularly highlighted as ongoing major concerns:

> Black and minority ethnic groups continue to express considerable disadvantages in the provision of mental health services because of the treatment which is appropriate to their need … . (Mental Health Commission, 1995: 85)

The Commision's concerns about mental health provision for black people continue to centre on matters which have been commented on in the previous five Biennial Reports of the Commission – that is:

- there are disproportionate numbers of patients of Afro-Caribbean origin detained under the Mental Health Act
- many Health Authorities do not address the needs of ethnic minority groups and
- ethnic monitoring (mandatory since 1 April 1995) is still implemented patchily. Many purchasers do not appear to include a requirement for ethnic monitoring in their contracts (Ibid.: 85–6).

There are, increasingly, welcome developments in the field of practice-related theory aimed at understanding and improving social work in the area of culturally-sensitive mental health. However concerns continue about the over-representation of black people within the compulsory mental health system, especially in relation to criminalisation and racial stereotyping (Fernando, Ndegwa and Wilson, 1998). Fernando (1991, 1995) has written specifically on mental health in a multi-ethnic society whilst, recently, Bhugra and others have explored the religious aspects to psychiatry and mental health (Bhugra *et al.*, 1997).

In the practice of the authors, psychoanalytic understanding has helped to illuminate some of the complex issues at work in both crisis mental health assessments, but also in longer-term situations. Clearly, whilst not all social workers are, or would hope or want to be, psychotherapists, it is hoped that, by sharing and reflecting on these ideas, continued improvement can be made to culturally-sensitive practice. What we are considering here, how-ever, is the common ground that exists between diverse areas of theory, and how psychoanalytic ideas hold some helpful clues for how to assist people who are in mental distress, without resorting to compulsory powers and, on the other hand, knowing when compulsory powers are finally necessary and how to use them in a humane way. It may be that some of the experi-ences felt and described by our clients may well be understandable within psychoanalytic descriptions but, for various reasons, social work action needs to be something other than offering psychoanalytic interpretations with a view to promoting insight.

Case examples

In the first example given below, we try to illustrate a situation where working towards insight was not possible, and the creation of a physically safe environment was paramount instead.

Note that not all the examples given below directly relate to approved social work. Broadening the scope allows us to highlight the range of issues involved and demonstrate the wide applicability of the concepts under discussion.

Example 1: Jimmy

Jimmy was a young white man from Scotland, living alone in London after coming over to work on the roads. He was arrested following a series of vicious attacks, which he perpetrated alone, on black people. He would calmly walk up to a black person in the street then, for no explicable reason, beat them senseless. On psychiatric examination, Jimmy was ascribed a diagnosis of paranoid schizophrenia. He was confined to a psychiatric hos-pital under section 37/41 of the Mental Health Act 1983. This gave the hospital power to treat him compulsorily but also meant that he could only leave the grounds with the permission of the Home Secretary. Social work with Jimmy took the form of developing a relationship with him in order to maintain a continuous perspective about his dangerousness and whether, or when, the Home Office might be advised that his illness had remitted sufficiently to allow him more freedom.

Comment

Jimmy could never explain why he had beaten up defenceless and innocent black people, except to say that they were 'bad' in some indefinable way. Overall, he felt that the world was a dangerous place, and that there were many plots and schemes afoot which rendered him extremely vulnerable. In his psychotic state of mind, he was therefore attempting to defend himself from a covert, and well organised conspiratorial attack. Jimmy's state of mind indicates that he was in a fragmented state as described in Kleinian thought 'externalising the internal confict ... evades the torturing cruelty of the internal objects' (Hinshelwood, 1989: 126).

Jimmy's persecutors were indeed his own split-off, dangerous impulses, which he had projected into his victims. Bion, a follower and exponent of Kleinian thought, describes how the mind in such a disordered, psychotic state, feels itself to be surrounded by 'bizarre objects' (Bion, 1967: 39) which are its own internal persecutors experienced externally. In sociological terms, it is perhaps of interest that Jimmy himself was from a dispossessed and powerless group, and was a little apart from the society in which he found himself. Jimmy required physical management and containment in order to keep himself and society in a safe position.

In terms of projective identification, it could be argued that there were two strands at work. The first strand was the sense in which Jimmy experienced his internal world as being out of control. His criminal actions evoked the intervention of the judicial process in the form of rigid and strict controls as applied by the Mental Health Act. The second strand was more localised and immediate in the sense that Jimmy's aggression could well have resulted in retaliation from members of his local community in which case those deemed 'bad' by Jimmy would have been acting in accordance with his psychotic images of them. Although 'insight' was not a primary goal for the social worker involved with Jimmy, a rapport was established between them. Working together with the multidisciplinary team it was possible, over time, to help Jimmy move to a group living situation where, although still under formal supervision, Jimmy was able to experience more freedom of movement.

A secondary function of psychoanalytic understanding and awareness is to help the social worker make sense of, and therefore survive, what often seem to be complex and dangerous delusions on the part of the client.

The above example illustrates the importance of psychoanalytic understanding. The following example illustrates the importance of action – in this case, in the context of youth and community work.

Example 2: the youth worker

A youth worker in a deprived inner-city area was working with a group of skinhead boys. The boys all lived on a local estate, known for its racist attacks. The youth worker happened to be Jewish. As the relationship developed with the boys, she became concerned, then angry, because of their continual reference to 'bloody Jews'.

Finally, the worker, who was in fact the daughter of Holocaust survivors, felt beside herself with rage and, without premeditation, said simply that she was Jewish. There was a few minutes' pause and a shocked silence from the boys. They then expressed disbelief.

'Are you Miss?' one of them said. They then began to ask her questions about Judaism, expressing as they did, some of the stock-in-trade beliefs that her parents had heard from their days in Central Europe before the Second World War, about believing that Jews sacrificed Christian children and drank their blood at Passover, for example. The worker was able to correct these misapprehensions.

At one point, one of the group confessed that they thought that 'Jews were different' and never would have believed that she was a Jew.

Comment

In his writings on group psychology, Jung warns of the dangers of 'mass psychology'. He believed that, by leading psychotherapy in Germany during the rise of Hitler, he could have counteracted some of the worst effects – particularly by ensuring that Jews were still allowed to practise psychotherapy when the Nazis tried to ban them from doing so (Jung, 1955, letters, 28 March 1934: 155). In this example, the youth worker was caught up in a perhaps more difficult confrontation, because it was between her, her own identity, her parents' identity (and their survival) and a group of potentially dangerous young men.

However she was able to confront them partly, if not wholly, because she had built up a relationship of trust with them, and through this was able to ameliorate their frightening, persecutory fantasies. She clearly ran a risk in this situation, being alone and with a group of potentially violent young men. In this case, the risk paid off, although if planning for such disclosures of personal identity it may be rather wiser to structure such groups with the assistance and presence of co-workers!

We have tried to explore practical issues of handling racism in social work from the perspective of the individual worker confronted by an individual lacking insight, together with the example of a volatile situation where insight was attained at some risk to the individual practitioner.

Unresolved racism at an institutional level can be destructive to individual workers and teams and result in catastrophe as in the following example.

Example 3: management in a multicultural environment

Mrs R was a social work manager. She also happened to be from Bangladesh. One day, she was attacked by a gang of boys in the street. Some of the boys were black, some were white. She was not physically injured, but was rather shaken up. Mrs R continued working and did not take any time off.

She had been having problems with a male member of her team. He tended to disrupt the team and was disliked by clients. One day, shortly after the attack, she could tolerate his behaviour no longer and informed him that she was going to start monitoring his work and performance. Immediately, the worker put in a grievance complaint, over Mrs R's head, to her manager, alleging that he had been subject to racist treatment. Mrs R's manager set the grievance procedure in motion, but, in the meantime, the worker refused to cooperate with the performance-monitoring exercise, claiming that his grievance was an appeal.

Mrs R sought the advice of her manager – a man – but could obtain no clear direction as to whether or not the worker's grievance constituted an appeal. She then checked with Personnel. Each personnel officer offered a different piece of advice. Meanwhile, the worker's behaviour deteriorated, and he became quite rude and insolent. Mrs R began to have sleepless nights, and found it hard to face going into work. She started to have flashbacks of her assault by the gang. To make matters more difficult, she was still continuing to try to be the dutiful Bengali mother and wife to her immediate and extended family – cooking, cleaning, washing and so on.

The grievance was finally heard, some three months after it was lodged, and was in fact rejected. Next day, over a minor matter, a further grievance was lodged. Mrs R now started to have headaches. Her work began to suffer, but she continued to go into work. She had never had time off work in 15 years' service. Then one day she collapsed at work, and was rushed to hospital. She died shortly afterwards of a stroke.

Comment

This example illustrates some of the pressures which people from ethnic communities can face, in a kind of complex interlocking weave, each pressure adding to the burden until the burden proves too great to bear. As in the first example, 'Jimmy', there is evidence here of the way in which discriminated groups are often pitted together in a destructive way. This is perhaps an example of projective identification at a societal and group level. The controlling group in society projects, into the controlled, or disaffected groups, the feelings and impulses which the controlling group does not wish to acknowledge, (through discriminatory housing or employment practices or policies, for example) so that these hostile feelings and impulses are acted out through racist attacks, interracial conflict and so on. In a management structure which is afraid of its own unconscious racism these elements will not be contained, and so workers will be encouraged to act them out against each other or against clients.

Returning to our consideration of the use of envy in Kleinian thought, which Klein originally referred to as the envy of the infant for the mother's breast and what it contained, it might be adduced that a worker could well feel envious of a manager and his or her position, especially if the manager is seen and experienced as being capable, as Mrs R was. The possibility of attacks based on envy is a very strong one. It is on that note that we now want to turn these reflections towards some considerations as to the significance of what could be referred to as attacks on difference, in ways described in the psychoanalytic context by Chasseguet-Smirgel (1985).

Example 4: the management committee

A community worker, employed by a management committee of local people from an estate, discovered that a key member of the committee held strongly racist views. Indeed he and his views were so unpleasant that other committee members were driven away. People were, after all, giving up their time voluntarily, so why should they be subject to his unpleasantness? The problem for the community worker was that the committee – including the racist – were his employers.

The community worker pondered how to deal with this problem. Another part of the community worker's role was to help develop the committee to be able to take charge of the project which was being set up. Thus the strategy adopted by the worker was to support and empower the more positive and forward-thinking members of the committee so that they did not leave, whilst also encouraging them to take the power they had as full committee members to vote against the racist member should they want to.

Eventually, the racist member became so disgruntled at continually being voted down that he walked out of a meeting in disgust one day, never to return.

Comment

There is an ethical issue here inasmuch as the community worker might be perceived to be imposing his own non-racist views on to the committee. However the worker was reassured in this by the number of members who felt that their fellow member's comments and attitudes to be so difficult and unpleasant that they were unable to work with him.

In political terms, this example illustrates the problem democracy has with dictators: a sufficiently charismatic dictator can be voted into power on the basis of a disempowering agenda: 'The state is aghast, a mirror-reflex of the personal ruler' (Jung, 1936: 92). Through persuasion and effort the worker, in this example, was able to use group processes to empower the group to reject racism.

Example 5: Gilles de la Tourette's syndrome

Gilles de la Tourette's syndrome is a psychiatric disorder characterised by involuntary tics, physical mannerisms, and occasionally the utterance of expletives, sometimes of a racist nature. In this example, the presentation offered by the client was so frightening and disordered that no hostel was prepared to accept him. He had been admitted to hospital for short stays, but did not need sustained inpatient treatment.

Following his discharge he lived on the streets for a short time, while the social worker desperately worked with a drop-in centre for homeless people which did not refuse him access as well as working educationally with a hostel for street-dwellers to help workers understand what this syndrome meant, including emphasising that this man's expletives were a sign of his inner distress rather than racism.

Comment

Social work with mental illness can take many forms. In this case, the worker had to suppress his own feelings of difficulty at this client's degree of difference, in order to help him find accommodation, and be supported through the process. This example also highlights the need for a range of provisions, with staff who understand the range and implications of mental disorder.

8 Drugs, alcohol and addictions

Introduction

The theme of this chapter relates to the extremely wide area now often referred to as substance use. Since addictive behaviours have also been described in relation to situations not involving chemical substances we have tried to broaden the scope of the chapter somewhat to include those areas since, with regard to the compulsion to repeat, some authors and clinicians use the term or ascription 'addictive personality' by which is meant a person who tends to become dependent in many areas of their lives. As with many psychiatric terms or situations, the difference may not be so vast between what many of us do, or how many of us are, as against those relative few who are referred for mental health attention.

The description 'substance use' is now often preferred because it remains a morally neutral description, whilst at the same time making no inappropriate distinctions between types of behaviour as might be the case if such terms as 'substance misuse', 'drug dependence', 'addiction', 'alcoholic', or more negative and condemnatory ascriptions such as 'junkie', 'dosser', 'wino' were used. Similarly, the use of the term 'substance use' allows a very broad interpretation of what is involved. Substance use can include the following substances:

- coffee and tea (caffeine)
- alcohol
- tobacco (nicotine)
- glue

- lighter fuel
- cleaning fluid
- illicit, non-prescribed drugs
- legal, but not prescribed, drugs
- prescribed drugs.

Substance use and the Mental Health Act 1983

Approved social workers are not permitted to use powers under the Mental Health Act 1983 to detain a person solely for reasons of dependency on drugs or alcohol, as clearly stated by section (3):

> Nothing in subsection (2) ... shall be construed as implying that a person may be dealt with under this Act as suffering from mental disorder, or from any form of mental disorder described in this section, by reason only of promiscuity or other immoral conduct, sexual deviancy, or dependency on alcohol or drugs.

Case example 1

A young woman had taken to her bed and refused to get up. She spent her time drinking cognac, and was getting through over a bottle per day. In assessment with an approved social worker and duty psychiatrist, she seemed low in spirits, but not clinically depressed. The duty psychiatrist contacted the consultant psychiatrist who regularly treated this woman.

The consultant felt that hospital admission would achieve very little, as she had been low in spirits for many years and hospital admission seemed to make no difference – if anything, it had sometimes made her more depressed. The woman agreed to consider, with the social worker, an alcohol treatment centre and, in the meantime, was monitored by a friend who called to see her daily. Despite calling back over the next few days, the approved social worker was unable to persuade the woman to agree to an alcohol programme. A further assessment visit was arranged with the duty psychiatrist, but no formal psychiatric symptoms could be elicited at all on that occasion. The young woman was rational, lucid and continued to express the point of view that she wanted to lie in bed and drink all day. She had private financial means and could afford it. The approved social worker and psychiatrist felt there was no more that either of them could do on that occasion.

Comment

Unlike in the example above, where behaviour of a psychotic nature has occurred, possibly as a result of drug or alcohol use, then use of the Mental Health Act could well be appropriate. Use of certain drugs – especially amphetamines – can result in feelings of paranoia, whilst withdrawal from heavy alcohol consumption can also give rise to feelings of panic and paranoia. If such feelings become overwhelming and place a person or others close to them at risk, then formal admission may be indicated, but based on the paranoid ideation, not on the addiction.

Case example 2

A young man of mixed racial heritage was arrested after slashing a seat in a tube train with a machete. On psychiatric examination, he was felt to be suffering from schizophrenia. Following drug treatment and several months in a psychiatric hospital – to which he had been transferred from prison – he was discharged. He lapsed from treatment and, after some weeks, was arrested following another incident of violence. He then told his doctors that he smoked cannabis regularly and frequently.

Over the next few months he was kept under close observation and, finally, his consultant did formulate the view that cannabis use did exacerbate this young man's paranoia since, when he did not smoke it, he remained rather well, even without antipsychotic drugs. As soon as he began to smoke cannabis, however, his paranoid symptoms became worse and, furthermore, he became quite dangerous.

Comment

In recent years debate has arisen over the term 'cannabis psychosis' in terms of its potential to justify racist overtreatment of people from black and ethnic minorities. Similarly, the chewing of Khat amongst Somali men has also evoked debate about the possibility, or not, of symptoms of psychosis. Wolff *et al.* (1990) report some evidence of short-lived psychotic reactions although, as Fernando observes, the diagnosis of cannabis psychosis is almost exclusively given to black people (Fernando, 1995, quoting McGovern and Cope, 1987).

In recent years, very heavy use of cannabis has been connected with foetal abnormality, and some recent work from the USA suggests that there may be long-term memory loss and dependency factors.

In the above example, the hypothesis about a connection between cannabis and paranoia was only arrived at after extensive observation of the young man concerned.

Substance use and the National Health Service and Community Care Act 1990

Prior to the implementation of the NHS and Community Care Act in April 1993, the care and treatment for people with problems associated with substance use was inconsistent and patchy to say the least. Medical treatment in terms of detoxification and withdrawal were the responsibilities of local health authorities, but were dependent on service users' cooperation. Furthermore, aftercare was a local authority responsibility but was not mandatory and very hazily enforced. Local councils made grants available to local drug and alcohol services, dependent on the humanitarian arguments which could be made by each agency on an individual basis. The authors have experience of situations prior to the NHS and Community Care Act in which people with drug and alcohol problems were neglected, discharged from psychiatric hospitals without any aftercare, or died on the streets, frozen solid, in winter. Kearney (1989) characterises a traditional view of drug-users as being 'mad, bad, and dangerous to know'.

Case example 3

A client who, for many years, had experienced problems accessing a social worker because of his propensity to violence and the fact that he had an alcohol problem was, under the new arrangements for community care, assessed for alcohol rehabilitation funding. Such was the depths of this man's previous record of violence that he had spent a considerable time in prison for carrying offensive weapons, such as long knives, and blackmail. On this occasion, however, he was accepted as being in need and funded at a local alcohol rehabilitation hostel. After two nights, he returned to the hostel drunk and threatening staff. He was evicted. He then came looking for the social worker who had made the community care assessment in order to beat him up, blaming him for the failure of services. This man did, indeed, smash up the office but succeeded in running away before the police arrived.

Comment

Such an incident requires perhaps quite complex understanding about human interaction. This man had received a service from the local authority for the first time in many years and, indeed, had received what he had asked for. The social worker had behaved correctly, made an appropriate assessment, and funding had been authorised by the budget-holder. At a formal level, everything had worked. From a psychoanalytic perspective, however, people experiencing addictions are struggling with massive, but unconscious, destructive urges.

Such destructive urges become acted out in cases such as this, especially where there is what Winnicott (1963) would describe as a 'good enough' object, which has shown some capacity to try to understand and make contact with the client. Indeed, the better the contact, in psychoanalytic terms, the more risk is run of acting out. The unconscious feelings which are felt as intolerable to the person, want to find a place and someone who can tolerate them.

If there is a sign in the external world that someone wants to know, and tolerate them, they emerge. At another level, this is a reason why people with severe personality disorders end up in prison – because it is only the concrete walls and iron bars of prisons which can tolerate and contain some of the unconscious and massively destructive forces at work which constantly seek expression.

The NHS and Community Care Act 1990, implemented in 1993, placed local authorities at the centre of matters, giving them the lead role in implementing community care. They were expected to engage in partnership with local drug and alcohol agencies, to plan community care jointly, be responsible for commissioning proper assessment arrangements for people with drug and alcohol problems, and to inspect and monitor services. The funding for this was to come out of the special transitional grant (STG), from budgets previously held by the DSS.

Controversy raged at the time about the amounts of the STG and how these were determined locally. The relevant and important issue here is that local authorities became responsible for people with drug and alcohol problems. Taken together with approved social worker's duties under the Mental Health Act, and the fact that people with mental health problems may also have problems associated with drug or alcohol use (or both), we can see that the mental health professional's role in general, and the approved social worker's role in particular, can become complex webs of responsibilities and judgements.

The Police and Criminal Evidence Act 1984

The Police and Criminal Evidence Act 1984 (PACE) adds yet another dimension to the potential complexity of the helping role in relation to work with substance use, especially since many people who are arrested will have experienced substance use as the precipitating cause – directly or indirectly – of their arrest. Under the PACE requirements it is a mandatory duty laid upon the police when questioning a person known or suspected to have mental health problems or be in some other way 'vulnerable', to have present an 'appropriate adult' as that person's representative. The appropriate adult must be an independent person, not the suspect's solicitor, who is able to take an active part in the police interview in terms of explaining what is said to them, helping them understand the nature of the interview, their rights and duties and so on.

As PACE has developed, some local authorities have begun to develop appropriate adult panels of volunteers who are on call to attend police stations, sometimes using financial support from schemes such as the Mental Illness Specific Grant. It is important, in the experience of the authors, for PACE workers to be properly trained in both PACE, mental health and, indeed, community care, since all these areas become operationalised when working in this area.

Case example 4

An approved social worker is called by the police to act as an appropriate adult for a young white man who was arrested for smashing milk bottles outside an old people's home.

He was drunk, and the police felt that there was something 'strange' about him (many police referrals come about in this way – a hunch or intuition from the arresting officer or duty sergeant). Under questioning, the young man confessed to having a drink problem – drinking several cans of strong lager a day. But he also said he was being hounded by a gang who were trying to kill him. The approved social worker was not sure how much of the man's story was fantasy and how much was reality – was he suffering a paranoid illness as well as alcoholism, for example? However, after making some enquiries on the telephone, the approved social worker discovered that the man had received previous psychiatric treatment and, indeed, had once been beaten up inexplicably. The young man said he was frightened to go back to his flat, and had smashed the milk bottles in desperation.

The young man agreed to admission to a detoxification unit. The police agreed not to pursue charges. The young man stayed in the unit, then went on to rehabilitation, and finally was rehoused.

Comment

This perhaps unusually successful outcome illustrates a number of points:

- The approved social worker and police had a sufficiently good working relationship as to trust each others' capacities and judgements.

- The police on duty knew – or suspected – enough about mental health problems to make an appropriate referral.
- The approved social worker had sufficient knowledge of alcohol, mental health and locality services to know with whom to speak, and how to make differential assessments about the respective needs for psychiatric assessment, alcohol detoxification and housing.
- The approved social worker did not make superficial judgements about the client's story.

Substance use and social work training

With the implementation of community care, the importance of training for social workers in substance use has come to be recognised.

The Central Council for the Education and Training of Social Workers (CCETSW) – the statutory regulatory body for social workers – publishes four guides to this: *Substance Misuse* (1992), *Alcohol Problems* (1993), *Alcohol Interventions* (1995), and *Substance Misuse: Designing Social Work Training* (1993). However, until recently, substance use/misuse training did not receive a high priority on social work training courses either pre- or post-qualification. These various reports emphasise that working with substance use needs to be recognised as part of the core social work task, and that there are a range of core values, knowledge and skills associated with this. In our experience, drug and alcohol agencies frequently observe and complain that social workers either do not know enough, are not prepared to engage with, or are not sufficiently alert to, the issues involved in substance use.

This applies to work with adults and children, since either group can be substance users, or be the parents of, or the offspring of, people who use drugs or alcohol.

Types of substance

It might be helpful to classify in a little more detail some of the effects, and the legal position, of the various drugs and substances which we have been discussing. Referring back to our list at the beginning of this chapter, we now take each substance in turn:

- **Caffeine** (found in coffee, tea, some soft drinks and other foods). In its pure form can be toxic. In diluted form (as in coffee and such like), can lead to palpitations, excitability and dependency. Legally available.

- **Alcohol.** Some medical debate has recently arisen over the possible positive effect of 'moderate' drinking. Heavy and consistent alcohol use over years can result in a number of illnesses and medical conditions ranging from damage to the brain, the liver, stomach, pancreas and heart. The difference between moderate and heavy has, up until recently, been 21 units per week for men and 14 for women (where one unit is one measure of alcohol). Alcohol is legally available to adults.
- **Nicotine** (found in tobacco). The effects of long-term cigarette smoking are now well attested. Recently, attempts have been made by smokers stricken with cancer or other associated illnesses to take cigarette companies to court. Legally available to adults.
- **Glue, lighter fuel and cleaning fluid** (now grouped together as 'solvents'). Also included in this group could be fire extinguishers, hair lacquer, nail varnish, typewriter correction fluid, paint stripper or paint thinner. The issue of solvent abuse, as it is now known, has emerged in recent years as a serious problem, especially for young people in relation to the legal availability of many of the substances just described.

    For example, since 1985 solvent abuse has killed an average of 117 people each year, over 70 per cent of whom have been under 20. The typical age onset is in the age range 11–17 (HMSO, 1995). Symptoms can include irritability, nausea, damage to the brain, liver, kidneys, bone marrow, delusions and hallucinations and, in extreme cases, sudden death which can occur uniquely at first exposure to the substance. In that sense, this is a serious, life-threatening matter.
- **Illicit, non-prescribed drugs.** These fall into three legal classifications, each with a maximum penalty for possession or for trafficking:

    - Class A: possession carries a maximum seven years' imprisonment plus an unlimited fine; trafficking, a maximum of life imprisonment plus an unlimited fine.

        Common drugs: cannabis oil, LSD, Ecstasy, heroin, morphine, methadone, opium, pethidine, cocaine/crack, magic mushrooms, PCP.
    - Class B: possession: a maximum of five years' imprisonment plus an unlimited fine; trafficking, a maximum of 14 years' imprisonment plus an unlimited fine.

        Common drugs: cannabis resin, marijuana, amphetamine, codeine, barbiturates.
    - Class C: possession: a maximum of two years' imprisonment plus an unlimited fine; trafficking, five years' imprisonment plus an unlimited fine.

        Common drugs: tranquillisers, distalgesics.

Apart from the problem of drug dependency, which can occur with all the above, and various physiological problems, other serious psychiatric problems can arise with the use of many of the drugs referred to, but especially the following:*

- Amphetamines/speed/whiz/bill/sulphate/pink champagne/ dexies (paranoia)
- barbiturates/barbs/sleepers/downers/yellow jacket/rainbow (depression)
- cannabis/dope/blow/grass/spliff/ganga/hash/weed/pot/joint/ shit (paranoia)
- cocaine/coke/snow/charlie (anxiety)
- crack cocaine/rock/wash/freebase/shit/base (agitation and irritability)
- Ecstasy/MDMA/adam/EXTC/white doves/love doves/disco burgers (manic-depressive psychosis, depression)
- LSD/acid/trips/tabs (schizophrenia).

- **Legal but not prescribed drugs.** It is not prohibited to possess anabolic steroids; indeed, these have been used to enhance performance in body-building. However, they too have been shown to become addictive and cause episodes of aggression and psychosis, quite apart from a range of physiological problems.
- **Prescribed drugs.** In recent years the problem of dependency upon prescribed medication, especially tranquillisers, has been recognised. This has stimulated some controversy, both in terms of the possible overuse of minor tranquillisers, especially for women, and in terms of the debate about the use of major tranquillisers in the treatment of schizophrenia. From a critical perspective, Breggin has written of what he describes as 'Toxic Psychiatry' (Breggin, 1993). He criticises what he sees as the vast overuse of tranquillising medication for psychiatric patients, women, children and homeless people, referring to it as 'suppressing the passion', and advocating instead more radical means including psychological alternatives and psychotherapy. However, Breggin is careful to warn that suddenly stopping any drug is dangerous, hence the movement amongst many self-help mental health service user groups to set up what are described as 'tranquilliser support groups' to assist in the process of withdrawal from medication. Clearly, where such medication might be prescribed by a

* With grateful acknowledgement to the Focus Drug Information Booklet, Nottingham Community NHS Trust and Nottingham Drugs Prevention Team. We also reproduce some street names of each drug, although these may vary from area to area.

psychiatrist relating to community supervision arrangements, any such withdrawal procedures might need to be checked out and full medical and/or legal advice given.

Case example 5

A middle-aged woman was receiving regular medication for her relapsing psychotic illness. One day her daughter consulted her GP who in turn consulted the social services department about a crisis. At a local squat, the woman had met a homeless man who had persuaded her to give up her medication and to accompany him on a journey to the East.

On visiting her flat, the two approved social workers,* a GP and the lady's daughter found all the furniture strewn carelessly into the middle of the road. Smoke was wreathing through the front door. Inside the flat, furniture was piled high and the approved social worker could hardly see for smoke. The floor was covered by several inches of water. In the kitchen, the middle-aged woman was heaping blankets on to a lit electric fire, the wires to which were trailing in the water.

At the sight of her daughter, the woman shrieked and grabbed her as if trying to pull her on to the fire. The approved social worker and her colleague restrained the woman, while the GP located the master fuse to switch off the electricity so that they were not all electrocuted. The police arrived, summoned in case the homeless man had been present and in case he too had needed either restraint or assessment.

Perhaps fortuitously, the homeless man had fled before the assessment team had arrived. Besides the police, the approved social workers summoned the fire brigade to ensure that the fire was put out and electricity supply rendered safe. The woman who had been the subject of the assessment was placed under section 2 for assessment. The presence of police and fire crew seemed to calm the situation down sufficiently so that she allowed herself to be conveyed to hospital in an ambulance. All the emergency services were needed, and the approved social workers' task involved the coordination of a complex range of issues and services.

Comment

Health and safety are crucial issues, but even the best of plans cannot always account for unforeseen circumstances. This was a very distressing situation

---

* Two approved social workers attended this assessment because, from the presentation, it had appeared that the homeless man might also have had mental health problems.

for the lady's daughter who had brought about the referral. However, had a referral not been made, the lady may well have been killed in a fire or by electrocution, as might well have been neighbours.

Types of intervention

Broadly speaking, intervention falls into four categories:

1   education to help make people aware of the problems associated with drug use and hopefully therefore prevent it (for example, work in schools to help children understand the dangers of getting involved with drugs);
2   helping children say 'no' to drugs;
3   work with parents to help them understand the pressures on children in relation to drug use;
4   treatment to minimise the harm associated with substance use (for example, recognising that, for some people, abstention is completely impossible due to the longevity of their habit, or other associated chronic social problems). This approach helps introduce other factors such as healthy diet, clean syringes and needle exchanges, in order to minimise the risks otherwise associated with substance use.

We referred above to the contribution psychoanalytic understanding might make to the issues associated with substance use. Rosenfield (1964) provides an extremely thorough evaluation of psychoanalytic writings on this subject, although noting that much work had been written up to 1945, but little after, possibly in recognition of the difficulties which drug and alcohol addiction present to treatment.

A number of variations of interpretation are offered within a psychoanalytic method but, essentially, the drug is understood as a kind of idealised object which the individual feels that they lack, but which at the same time – paradoxically – is felt to be absolutely destructive. This is expressed in the saying from Alcoholics Anonymous that 'one drink is too many; a thousand not enough'.

Indeed Bateson's (1973) view of one of the prime reasons for the success of Alcoholics Anonymous is precisely because it recognises that it requires a power greater than the self to rescue the self from alcohol which is, by its nature, more powerful than the individual; hence the idea in AA that the alcoholic surrenders him or herself to God 'as we understood him' (Alcoholics Anonymous *12 Steps*).

Substance use and risk

It is not always, or not only, the chemical substance used which induces risk factors. Other risk factors which come into play are:

- developing a criminal record – a serious concern for young people and their future, or older people who risk losing their jobs
- health factors associated with the supply of substances – for example, their purity (or lack of it) and the fact that the impurities can do far more harm than the pure substance itself
- needing ever greater quantities of the substances – therefore developing an expensive lifestyle which, given the difficulties in obtaining the substance and the aftereffects of its consumption, make it increasingly difficult to finance
- health factors associated with the ingestion of the substances – for example, contracting HIV/AIDS by sharing dirty needles, contracting hepatitis B through contaminated blood
- contingent risks associated with the aftereffects of ingestion – for example, sexual disinhibition making a person more vulnerable to exploitation or placing them at risk of unprotected sex; depression, agitation or jealousy which can increase the risk of suicide or homicide; carelessness which can give rise to serious accidents.

Case example 6

A man with a diagnosis of schizophrenia subsequently developed a heroin habit. He kept in touch with his social worker intermittently, largely to try to obtain either money directly, or to ask for money. One day, the client revealed that his flat had been taken over and he could not stay there. The man who had taken over his flat bullied him. Things had been OK at first – they had helped each other out and helped each other get drugs. Now, and as a result of his mental health problems complicated by heroin use, this client had nowhere to live, was not eating properly, and was using dirty needles, exemplifying the risk to self discussed above.

With the assistance of the housing department and the police, the social worker was able to help this man get back into his flat and eventually get him rehoused.

Comment

The social work ideal of 'empowerment' can sometimes become very blurred in trying to help people cope with chaotic lifestyles. The man needed urgent, practical help to bring his life back into a manageable shape so that he could then have the opportunity to live safely, survive, and think about empowerment. It could have been very easy for the services to wash their hands of him at his point of crisis because he had somehow 'got himself into that mess', whilst using that as a rationalisation for their underlying feeling that at that point in his life he had indeed become 'mad, bad and dangerous to know'.

Case example 7

An example of a situation which involved many issues in this chapter, but also relates to our discussions of risk to both the self and others started with a referral from a day hospital to the duty approved social worker. A patient had discharged himself the previous evening, but had been given an appointment the following day for an interview at a day hospital. He had not kept his day hospital interview. Somewhat efficiently, the day hospital had telephoned the client who said that he was not going to the day hospital; he was going to stay indoors and drink himself into oblivion. He ended the call abruptly, saying that he wanted to die. The client lived in a hostel. The duty approved social worker contacted the hostel warden who had not seen the client all day. In fact, he was not sure whether the man was in or not. Because of the referral from the day hospital, and the possible level of risk involved, the approved social worker agreed to visit. Given the facts that neither was he sure the man was in, together with the on-site availability of a warden, the approved social worker felt that precautions such as obtaining police assistance, or even the presence of a doctor were unnecessary.

On arrival at the hostel, the approved social worker was taken upstairs to the fourth floor to the client's room. There was no answer to their knock on the door.

As it happened, the warden had a key and, after receiving no reply to their shouts, he opened the door.* On entering the room, they saw the client lying on his bed. He had his eyes closed, and might have been asleep, except that, in one hand he had a can of lighter fuel, in the other hand was a cigarette and, on his bedside table, there was an opened can of strong lager.

The approved social worker explained who he was and why he was there. The man opened his eyes and, at first, was willing to talk. He agreed that he had rung the hospital and acknowledged that he was depressed because he saw no point in continuing to live. After a few moments, the warden asked if he could be excused, as he had to attend to other matters in the hostel. Seeing

---

* It will be recalled that, under section 115 of the Mental Health Act, the approved social worker has a right to enter and inspect a premises, unless entry is refused.

no health or danger threat, the approved social worker expressed his consent. It was only after the warden left that the client started to become hostile and threatening. He intermittently sniffed at the lighter fuel bottle, sipped from his can of lager and puffed at his cigarette. He began to speak of jumping out of the window (it was the fourth floor, it will be recalled) and, when the approved social worker moved to stand by the window to prevent this, the man said that when he decided to go, he would take the approved social worker with him.

Fortunately, the approved social worker had a mobile telephone. As the man slipped in and out of consciousness, he was able to dial 999 and ask for urgent police assistance. Fortunately, the police arrived quite quickly but not before the client had managed to stand and there had been a few moments of wrestling by the window. The first action they took was to remove the danger of an explosion by taking away the man's butane canister. They then removed to safety the number of knives that the approved social worker had now noticed around the room. The client once more became quite agitated and hostile, and needed to be restrained by the police.

While this was going on, the approved social worker made contact with the duty psychiatrist who fortunately was able to attend quickly.

There was then some discussion about use of section 4. As indicated above, no section of the Act should be used solely for purposes of dealing with drug or alcohol addiction. However, this man was an active suicide risk – possibly as a result of agitation produced as a result of the combination of solvent and alcohol misuse. Furthermore, no other doctor was available, and this certainly seemed to be an emergency. The approved social worker and the doctor agreed that section 4 was acceptable, and the client was conveyed to hospital.

Comment

In one sense the approved social worker could be said to have disregarded health and safety procedures; yet at the same time, this man, at the outset of their meeting, provoked no threat. Furthermore, every approved social worker needs to make a judgement about what constitutes an interview in an 'appropriate manner' which also involves some attempt to conduct an interview in as humane and ordinary way as possible. When going to this interview the approved social worker had no way of knowing that this man was as unpredictable as he clearly turned out to be. These considerations illustrate some of the many risks approved social workers run in the course of their duties. This particular worker was fortunate to escape with his life.

Other addictions

Rosenfield (1964) connects the addiction to food with drug addiction in terms of unresolved conflicts about infantile feeding at the breast. This is a largely Kleinian approach (Melanie Klein's works spanning the years 1921–63 are the most significant achievement in psychoanalytic literature after the Freud/ Jung dyad). Some other key addictions which have been described subsequently, more in terms of compulsive behaviour patterns, are addictions to sexuality, paedophilia, gambling, shoplifting and arson. The UCH *Textbook of Psychiatry* refers to the last three as 'disorders of impulse control' (Wolff *et al.*, 1991). Commonalities between all addictions and disorders of impulse control are such trends as a compulsion to repeat, the hopelessness of willpower and the centrality of the compulsive act irrespective of all other considerations – moral or practical.

It remains the task of each practitioner or clinician to resolve in his or her own mind what are the best, most efficacious, and most plausible tools which can be employed to ensure safety for the client, their close relatives, friends or carers (if there are any) and the public at each point of referral. It is hoped that these notes might serve as useful signposts in an impossibly difficult area in which to navigate.

9 Dangerousness, suicide and homicide

Introduction

The cluster of concepts contained in any consideration of dangerousness, suicide and homicide is at once incredibly wide, difficult to define and all-encompassing, yet at the same time, form the core of so much public alarm about mental health that it seems inevitable that they be considered together. It is this public alarm, followed by a number of official inquiries, that has led to much of the legislative change driving the increased community policing of the person deemed mentally ill that we are presently witnessing. Public alarm may be a recognition of genuine concern. A number of murders have been committed by people suffering from a mental illness. Mental hospitals have been closed. Whether the latter has created the space for the former may be a matter for debate. Public alarm about mentally ill people may also be a 'moral panic' into which society can evacuate its own negative and unwanted projections.

The correlation of mental illness with dangerousness does a conceptual violence to mental illness and dangerousness, as well as turning service users, clients or patients into frightening ogres who need to be feared. The testimony from service users is that they want their distress to be understood and for their aspirations to be valued. Breggin (1993) in his book *Toxic Psychiatry* makes this point, as does the earlier independent film made by service users, *We're Not Mad, We're Angry*. Empowerment and user participation are dealt with elsewhere in this book.

With reference to the issue of dangerousness it might be helpful to determine what the reality might be between, on the one hand, the wild anxieties of those who are troubled by the dangerousness of mentally ill people, as opposed to many mentally ill people themselves who feel maligned and misunderstood.

The Report of the Confidential Inquiry into Homicides and Suicides by Mentally Ill People (1996) closely analysed 39 cases of homicide between the periods of July 1992–January 1994 and September 1994–March 1995, and 240 cases of suicide between June 1993–December 1994. Although it is impossible to replicate here all the findings from this important report, there are three interesting observations to make. The first one is the finding which connects injury to self with injury to others, thus:

> Self-injury and aggression to others are frequently found together in the same patients. It is evident that the needs of both groups are very similar to each other and to the needs of other people with mental illnesses and mental disorders. (Ibid.: 56)

This idea indicates that there are elements of commonality between suicide and homicide – or harm to self and others – which need to be considered when addressing dangerousness.

The second relates to the assessment of risk: 'It is unrealistic to expect that every homicide or suicide is preventable' (ibid.: 64). This connects with a theme found in the Department of Health report, *The Prevention of Suicide* (Jenkins *et al.*, 1994), that, although suicide may not be absolutely preventable, good clinical practice can help reduce the likelihood of it occurring. Indeed, a Health of the Nation target is to reduce suicide rates by 15 per cent by the year 2000.

The report emphasises, nevertheless, that there are a number of steps that can be taken to minimise the risk of suicide or homicide, including:

- defined areas of accountability for each profession
- tackling non-compliance with medication
- training for staff in risk assessment
- improving and monitoring opportunities for patients and staff to have one-to-one contact
- adequate levels of staff and training for members of the multi-disciplinary team
- good communication and effective inter-agency work
- training for all staff in the provision of the Mental Health Act 1983
- the provision of sufficient in-patient beds and a pleasant therapeutic environment
- involving families in the treatment and care of their mentally ill relatives
- an appropriate range of local services for mentally ill people to interact with voluntarily and positively
- more research into the treatment of people with severe personality disorders
- mental health professionals to be more aware of the unsettling effects of

change on people's lives and be more aware of risk factors at times of change (e.g. holiday times, leaving hospital, changing address, and so on). (*Report,* 1996: 64–9).

In terms of the question of the comparative dangerousness of mentally ill people, this report notes that of an average 500 homicides per year, less than 100 perpetrators have been designated as legally abnormal, leading to the observation that 'there is a small but significant risk of violence by mentally ill people, notably those with psychotic disorders, particularly schizophrenia' (ibid.: 82). On the other hand, Hafner and Boker (1973) in their study concluded that people with schizophrenia were 100 times more likely to kill themselves than others.

Some other specific elements highlighted by the *Report* in relation to its review of homicides by mentally ill people are that most homicides were committed by men; the victim was known to the offender in three-quarters of cases, whilst in half the cases the victim was a family member or lover.

Puerperal psychosis

In considering the literature and research on homicide one finding of particular relevance for social workers working in child protection settings is that of a raised incidence of homicide by women suffering endogenous depression, whose victims were their own children. This most commonly occurs in the albeit rare cases of puerperal psychosis following the birth of an infant (estimated officially at one in 500 deliveries although a research review by Lucas (1994) places the prevalence somewhat higher). Some key points to note in relation to puerperal psychosis are as follows:

- It is most commonly found in mothers with a past personal or family history of mental illness.
- It usually develops within the first two weeks of delivery, but not often within the first two days.
- It can recur in a further pregnancy (the risk of this is 15–20 per cent of probabilities).
- Puerperal psychosis must be distinguished from postnatal depression. The former is a psychosis, occasioning a disruption of thinking and feeling, the latter is a neurosis sometimes called the 'baby blues' but is not a severe, life-threatening condition.

A typical presentation of puerperal psychosis is one of confusion and agitation, followed by delusional beliefs or thoughts about the patient's self, family or infant. It is because these delusional beliefs might cause the mother to harm her baby that intervention and assertive treatment might be necessary. For example, the mother might imagine that her baby will become enslaved to the devil if it lives and that it is therefore preferable to kill the baby – and for the mother to take her own life too – thus going to God and Heaven instead of staying in an evil world. In such a scenario, a mother might seek to hide or flee from social workers or doctors who could easily be seen as allies of the devil. In a case such as this, it would therefore be important for social workers to be fully aware of, and not shy away from using, provisions under section 135 of the Mental Health Act 1983 to search for and remove patients. This section of the Act empowers an approved social worker to apply to a magistrates' court in order to obtain a warrant which authorises a police constable to enter a premises, if needs be by force, in order to assess a person, and if necessary remove them to a place of safety.

Should steps to avert a child's death fail, a disposal open to a court is a finding of infanticide (Infanticide Act 1922, amended 1938). This allows a court to recognise circumstances of diminished responsibility on the part of the mother, leading to an order for probation or hospital treatment.

Managing dangerousness

Much of the research and literature published on homicide and suicide has been carried out by colleagues in psychiatry. One exception is Prins' *Offenders, Deviants or Patients* (1995). This is a wide-ranging and comprehensive analysis of issues relating to mental health and offending from a criminological and social work perspective. Prins makes the point that 'not all mentally disordered offenders are dangerous and that not all dangerous offenders are mentally disordered' (ibid.: 229). There is a context to 'dangerousness', and, used carelessly, 'dangerousness' means very little. In relation to daily social work practice, when we ask 'Is someone dangerous?', or think to ourselves, 'Is this a dangerous situation?', we are perhaps thinking more concretely about violence, because violence is how dangerousness is acted out.

Violence is frightening to social workers because, apart from the associated danger, it is not something that they consider as part and parcel of the job. This may be an increasingly questionable assumption given, as observed above, the increasing role they have in terms of policing – whether those policed are people with mental health problems, or children (or their parents) in need. Apart from policing those clients known to them, there are also the aspects of assessing those not known to them, but referred to social services – sometimes assessing a person who does not want to be assessed.

It is that sense social workers have of forcing themselves upon someone, or intruding into their lives, that can stimulate resentment which is manifested as violence – even if the assailant feels that his or her violence is carried out in self-defence. Brown *et al.* (1988) and Norris (1990) offered some preliminary investigations into social workers at risk (the former), and violence against social workers (the latter).

In the *Report of the Confidential Inquiry* (1996) notifications of eight suicides committed by social workers are recorded. As a matter of interest, this compares with 28 for consultant psychiatrists, 14 for 'other medical staff', 20 for nurses and community psychiatric nurses, 7 for psychologists, 2 for day centre workers, and 6 for 'others'. Amongst the population as a whole, vets and farmers have particularly high indices of suicides, followed by pharmacists and medical practitioners (Jenkins *et al.*, 1994). It will be recalled that a number of social workers have been murdered attempting to perform their duties, most in mental health settings. Regrettably, it was only after some of these incidents that changes in working practices, improving the health and safety of workers, were put in place. Examples of this are the introduction of entry-phones and enhanced office security following the murder of Isobel Schwarz, and the provision of mobile telephones and recognition of the need for approved social workers to be accompanied by colleagues or police, following the murder of Norma Morris.

Managing violence

In working out a scheme for the effective management of violence, one way of understanding might be to differentiate first between violence as a deliberate act and violence which is contingent. The difference here is that violence as a deliberate act will be violence acted out by an aggressor against a worker, whereas contingent violence will occur as part of a process of involvement. We will illustrate the difference by example.

Case example 1: violence as deliberate act

A client developed a grudge against a worker. This grudge began as verbal abuse and progressed to threats, before manifesting as an actual assault. The grudge might have arisen for a number of reasons: the client might have been denied a service or might have developed a psychotic delusional belief about the worker.

Case example 2: violence as contingent

In seeking to ensure the safe process of a mental health assessment, a worker enlisted the assistance of police and ambulance personnel. Following assessment and the decision that the client ought to be taken into hospital against their will, the client tried to flee, then when restrained, lashed out and hit the worker.

Comment

It is helpful to separate out violent assaults in this way as it helps depersonalise the feelings aroused by an assault – which we go on to explore below.

Trying to understand the notion of contingency can help when planning intervention in situations involving risk. Seeing some actions in terms of deliberation might also help plan for safety in situations where individual workers are targeted by challenging clients who might be extremely difficult to manage, and who present themselves as 'dangerous'. The problem with the idea of deliberate harm lies in the area of personality disorder: someone who targets another might be subject to psychotic delusions about that person (that they are controlling the client's life by means of telepathy, for example); alternatively, the aggressor might be suffering from a severe personality disorder. In such a situation, or in any situation of direct threats or targeting, a full medical, psychiatric and social assessment is necessary in order to ascertain whether formal and compulsory intervention is needed.

Case example 3: managing threats

An office was being bombarded with telephone calls from a client making abusive threats of a sexually explicit nature. The police were alerted and monitored the calls, included taping long and offensive messages. Some of the messages contained material which indicated the possible presence of a mental disorder, although this could not be conclusive. The office staff were extremely frightened and alarmed. The police and the approved social worker conferred and considered the possibility of forcing entry to the caller's flat, using a section 135 warrant, and assessing him for compulsory admission to hospital.

While these deliberations took place, the messages became more directly threatening, and it was decided that the police had sufficient evidence that he was making threats to kill. They then arrested the caller at a time pre-arranged with the approved social worker, who was available at the police station with two section 12-approved doctors. A mental health assessment took place at the police station, and the caller was found to be suffering from a schizophrenic illness requiring detention in hospital under section 3 of the Mental Health Act 1983. Criminal charges were not pursued. The patient was successfully treated and discharged home after some months in hospital.

Comment

This example illustrates the importance of, and the need for, police and approved social workers to be able to work together. In this instance, it enabled a man who was seriously ill to receive treatment which he needed. It also prevented a potentially serious situation of harm being caused to members of the public, as well as stopping the office workers – who were female – being the target of sexual harassment.

Nevertheless, formal intervention on the part of social or medical services do not always resolve themselves so positively, as the following example shows.

Case example 4: the force of law

A client targeted a worker because he identified the worker as being the prime cause of his being hospitalised against his will. The client assaulted the worker in the street and was arrested. On release from prison, the threats to the worker resumed.

The client was assessed by an approved social worker and doctors, but was not found to be suffering from a mental disorder within the terms of the Mental Health Act. Following this assessment, the client's threats resumed. Finally, an injunction was obtained, and the client's threats desisted.

Comment

The worker in this case was forced to resort to legal measures to seek to ensure his own safety. He was supported by his department in this, although there have been other cases where social service departments have refused to offer such support and workers have been forced to leave their posts. The client in this case was able to understand the consequences had he acted against the injunction and, indeed, the formal power of the court perhaps represented a form of psychological containment which he lacked in himself. In the instance of the mental health assessment, it is important to note that detention under the Mental Health Act 1983 is not dependent on a patient being a danger to himself or others (as frequently misquoted as being necessary). The important factors are that detention is shown to be necessary in the 'interests of the patient's health and safety, or the safety of others'.

Dangerousness as such is not mentioned in the Act. The Act does refer to 'psychopathic disorder' and, in section 3 (2) (b), proscribes the application for admission in terms of treatment being likely to alleviate or prevent a deterioration in the patient's condition and admission is necessary for the health and safety of the patient or the protection of others. This can present severe problems in the management of people with psychopathic conditions or severe personality disorders. In practice it often means that such patients are denied access to services until, and unless, they commit a serious offence or harm themselves to the extent of needing hospitalisation. Prins discusses these issues, commenting on the usefulness or otherwise of the concept of psychopathy. His rather tentative conclusions, based on consultation with a range of colleagues is that there is a need to set up specialised units for treating people with diagnoses of psychopathic disorders, especially in prisons and special hospitals (Prins, 1995: 137).

Stalking

Stalking or targeting can arise as a result of a particular grudge against an individual worker's action. Alternatively, stalking of a famous personality can be a result of a schizophrenic illness on the part of the stalker.

The stalker might have psychotic delusions about the person who is the object of their stalking for some imagined rebuff or imagined involvement.

The mass media has brought stalking into particular prominence in the eyes of the public; likewise, through the same mass communications, stalkers obtain a ready means of fame and notoriety – which may be attractive to them. Approved social workers and others involved in intervention in such matters may need to be particularly alert to the range of legal powers open to them and remember that effective and early intervention can sometimes save lives.

In this regard, it is important to note that The Protection from Harassment Act 1997 was specifically drafted to protect against stalking. It makes such actions as 'harassment and similar conduct' a criminal offence.

Clinical syndromes

In general terms, the clinical syndromes to which workers need to pay special caution with regard to risk factors associated with dangerousness, suicide or homicide are: paranoid schizophrenia, bipolar affective disorder (manic depressive psychosis), morbid jealousy, erotomania, severe personality disorder and psychopathy.

Social work and violence

Returning to our attempts to try to analyse the actual management of violence and focus on this issue in relation to social work we might go on to postulate four stages which need to be addressed by organisations and individual workers within them. These are discussed below.

Stage 1: prevention and avoidance

This includes:

- formulating and adhering to health and safety rules and policies
- installation of entryphones if appropriate
- adequate screens and protection for reception staff
- comprehensive history-taking, including past incidents of aggression
- passing on full information to colleagues when making referrals
- visiting in pairs where a client is not known, or when known to have a history of aggression
- alarm buttons in interview rooms (and adequate measures for responding to alarms and crises within offices – not only is it pointless but it is actively dangerous to have an alarm go off with no one responding to it!)
- use of mobile telephones for staff in dangerous environments
- good working relationships with police
- workers to sit between the client and door when interviewing clients, to prevent becoming 'boxed-in'.

Stage 2: de-escalation

Prevention and avoidance will not always work. It is important, therefore, to train staff in techniques for de-escalation. These might include helping staff:

- be able to keep calm when unforeseen circumstances occur
- not to panic
- talk quietly to a client who might be shouting
- remove themselves rapidly from a situation which is heading out of control
- not to try to be heroic, but to think of safety and avoidance as priorities.

Stage 3: management

Should de-escalation not be possible, staff need to have some clues as to how to manage themselves in a violent situation. Primarily this will mean:

- removing themselves from the situation or assailant

- asking for help
- protecting themselves as a priority and
- protecting the client if possible – although this will be a fine judgement.

On one occasion, one of the authors found himself alone with a client who was intermittently drinking alcohol, sniffing lighter fluid, and smoking cigarettes and who broke off from these pursuits to try to climb out of the fourth-storey window in order to throw himself to the ground, and take the author with him. Fortunately, the dilemma about how heroic to be or not was resolved by the arrival of the police. However, these are issues that we will not be prepared for if – or when – they happen, unless we think about them in advance. Some agencies have explored the use of physical techniques of 'breakaway training' in offering staff practical ways and means of escaping from violent situations. In special hospitals and secure units this is linked with appropriate training in 'control and restraint' for nursing staff.

Stage 4: aftercare and follow-up

Should stages 1–3 have passed, and we, or a member of our team, have been subject to an assault, it is important to have adequate policies and procedures in place for aftercare and follow-up. This might include automatic entitlement to time off work, counselling and debriefing. It is common for people who have experienced assault to blame themselves, so this is an area which needs to be addressed. It is also common for the full emotional impact not to emerge for some time – depending on the seriousness of the assault. Some people might find a torrent of verbal abuse as frightening as a physical attack. Conversely, some clients can offer quite frightening styles of verbal abuse. The Woodley Team Report (1995: 175) recommends that 'all health and social services providers have in place a plan of action for unexpected death and other untoward incidents', drawing this recommendation from *Disasters: Planning for a Caring Response* (HMSO, 1991).

Post-traumatic stress disorder

A single traumatic event can give rise to post-traumatic stress disorder, which is now a recognised clinical condition. Repeated traumatic events, or events which are not properly worked through can create chronic post-traumatic stress disorder, which is the term generally used to describe 'burnout'. The UCH *Textbook of Psychiatry* (Wolff *et al.*, 1991) offers the following criteria for post-traumatic stress disorder:

(1) The person has experienced a stressful event that is outside the range of usual human experience and would be markedly distressing to almost everyone.

(2) The event is being re-experienced in vivid dreams, intrusive recollections and flashbacks, usually in response to some triggering stimulus. Illusions and short-lived hallucinatory experiences also occur.

(3) The person avoids the stimuli which could be reminiscent of the disaster, leading to numbness, unresponsiveness and withdrawal.

(4) The person experiences increased arousal which was not present before the event. This includes difficulty in going to sleep or staying asleep; irritability or outbursts of anger; difficulty in concentrating; hypervigilance and an exaggerated startle response. Guilt about survival and memory impairment may also be present. (UCH, 1991: 189–90)

These criteria are reproduced in full because social workers may well recognise elements of themselves or their clients in this vivid clinical description. In this respect, it is well worth remembering health and safety legislation. Within the terms of the Health and Safety at Work Act 1974, employers have a general duty to ensure so far as is reasonably practical, the health, safety, and welfare of their employees – a 'duty of care'. Conversely, employees have a duty to take care and observe an organisation's rules and regulations. We have a duty to ourselves and each other to survive and help each other to survive. With the increasing demands made upon us we perhaps need to be ever more vigilant about this duty. This may need to be a personal and organisational imperative rather than a legislative one. It is a little known fact that assaults against social workers are not centrally recorded by the Health and Safety Executive since they are deemed 'not reportable' under the RIDDOR Regulations (1995) pertaining to the reporting of injuries, diseases and dangerous occurrences.

Personal values

Violence may be a difficult issue for social workers because they perceive themselves as being there to 'help' people, and physical attack comes then as a shock to their senses and their bodies. They are not at all prepared for it, either as a concept, or as an actuality. However, given the increase in the role of statutory intervention, clients may feel it is their right to defend themselves if their person is under attack; in the client's perception, a violent response may be a legitimate means of self-defence. This may not be easy for social workers to digest or stomach, but it highlights the need to be aware of where the profession stands on issues of liberty, self-defence and violence. This should be done before an incident occurs, because, once it does, in the heat of the moment, the worker's thinking, rational processes will not be working too well and he or she may freeze and not know what to do.

According to Gandhi 'Truth and non-violence are as old as the hills'. Certainly the origins of violence are ancient, as is our struggle to contain its worst manifestations. Explanations for violence which we each adopt might be based as much on our own predilections and world-view as on any objective or scientific explanation. Do we, for example, think of the human race as inherently in conflict and at war as, say, a behavioural psychologist might, or do we understand violence as a result of economic materialism in, say, a Marxian mode; or combine such a viewpoint and include psychodynamic explanations, as Fromm (1977) proposed in his monumental *The Anatomy of Human Destructiveness*? In his later work, Freud became preoccupied with issues of human conflict in his *Civilization and its Discontents* (1930). Such philosophical problems, including the riddle of why three world religions emanating from the same source have barely been able to live in peace since their respective creations are considered by Gaarder in the more recent *Sophie's World* (1996). Although it may be considered that such deliberations are not directly relevant to the subjects of dangerousness, suicide and homicide under consideration here, in terms of ideas of reference found in schizophrenia, both grandiosity and pseudophilosophy can often be found in great measure. They can have serious effects when acted out. In relation to social workers, if their own personal values have not reflected on some of these themes, they can be taken off guard as in the following example.

Case example 5: what shall I do?

A worker was attacked on the steps of his office by a psychotic client who repeatedly tried to beat him about the head. The worker protected himself as best he could by holding up his briefcase. As he did so, he shouted at the client to stop what he was doing otherwise he, the client, would get himself into trouble. During the incident the worker's mind was awash with a vast array of thoughts and options including:

- Should I try to hit back?
- Should I try to run away?
- Should I try to get back in the building?
- What do the crowd collecting around us think? Whose side are they on?
- Why are my colleagues not helping me? (A group of colleagues had gathered and were standing watching the events.)
- What are my rights if I hit back?

- This client is mentally ill – I need to keep him here so that help can come.
- If this goes on much longer I might die.
- What about my committment to non-violence?

Comment

In this example, there was an element of being frozen not only because the event was unexpected, but also because there was a conflict of personal values. At the same time, because the worker retained some presence of mind, he knew better than to run off and risk the client following him and both then being away from a potential source of help.

Gandhi (1927) admitted that, in all likelihood, his philosophy of non-violent passive resistance would not have worked against Hitler, whilst history is replete with other examples of people committed to non-violence being overwhelmed by forces outside their control. In light of continuing social work deaths – approved social worker Jenny Morrison was killed in 1998 while undertaking an after-care visit to a mentally ill client – social work departments must ensure that they have clear guidelines and operational policies on matters relating to health, safety and violence. This includes the identification of risk factors as well as what to do after an incident has taken place. It is not a traditionally accepted principle that social workers should learn basic self-defence, although this may be something to be considered as a last resort. Certainly nursing staff have access to courses in 'control and restraint' to enable them to deal effectively and safely with violent patients. It is arguable whether social workers should have access to similar opportunities.

10 Aspects of understanding

Introduction

Social work makes extreme and intense demands on us as practitioners. Clients make us feel despair, anger, frustration, sadness, failure. How do we cope with these feelings? How do we take care of ourselves?

One way of taking care may be to do just that. Take care not to become too involved; to become rigidly professional; to give just enough and nothing more; to take longer holidays; to attend lots of courses; to limit client contact; to reduce or 'rationalise' office and duty hours. 'Burnout' is a common phenomenon amongst members of the caring professions and has received considerable attention because of its destructive nature.

The combined effect of these various factors is, in one way or another, to deprive the client of ourselves. This may be what some of our clients want. However, is there another way of taking care of ourselves so as not to collude with some of the more destructive forces in our work? Is there a way to understand these difficulties and enable us to feel nourished and creative in what we do?

We can view these processes structually – see our difficulties in the light of our roles as members of a system. This is helpful, especially for workers in institutions. Another way may be to accept the feelings within us and use them as gateways to greater understanding. Used in this way, our feelings about our clients may act as a means of communication rather than as a hindrance.

Projective identification

A way of seeing a client and social worker interacting in this manner exists most clearly in the psychoanalytic concept of projective identification.

As an experience, projective identification can be found described in the clinical work of Freud and Jung. It was first described as a workable concept by Melanie Klein in her paper, 'Notes on Some Schizoid Mechanisms' in 1946. To understand the theory of projective identification, it is necessary to see feelings and emotions as part of the self. They can be experienced unconsciously as either attacking and persecutory or, alternatively, as rewarding and benevolent. Either of these sensations can be so overwhelming that, instead of being able to accept that they belong to oneself, the individual experiences the unconscious demand to project them out into someone else, thereby locating the centre of anxiety externally rather than internally. These feelings are projected onto others, but since they are nevertheless part of oneself, one still retains control over them; thus one is still identified with them. In this way, feelings become ways of manipulating other people unconsciously; other people become the bearer of one's own worst and best feelings.

Projective identification differs from projection in terms of degree. In projection, we may invest others with attributes and feelings that in reality are our own. In projective identification this becomes actually experienced by the other as an emotion inside them – something which may be quite strange to them and certainly difficult to control. Klein saw the origins of this process as lying in the earliest stages of infancy, where the infant's personality is disorganised and unintegrated, but liable to feel very powerful emotions. The infant puts these feelings into its mother in order to feel safe. It has two effects: the expulsion of 'bad things', and the creation of the sense of unconscious control over the mother. In later life these mechanisms are then repeated in our relationships with others.

Thus, we as social workers feel despair because the clients cannot – they are permeated with despair but, if they feel it at all, they would be overwhelmed by it. We feel anger at the client who feels inadequate and afraid, probably of his or her own anger. We fail the clients who are afraid of their failure. Like one of Laing's knots, the list and the variations are endless.

Case example 1

A young schizophrenic man lives at home with his mother and father. His mother spends her time being worried and exhausted by her son. His father absents himself, wanting nothing to do with his son whom he regards as a failure. The son spends his days either wandering the streets or sleeping in bed until all hours. His illness takes the form of delusions about being persecuted and haunted.

In this family there is a complex group process at work. The social worker experiences this in the form of helpless frustration occasioned by the schizophrenic's mother, which causes the social worker to flee the household in despair and exhaustion.

Comment

One dynamic that the example above highlights is the way in which the client's mother's concern is so strongly felt and expressed that it deeply affects the social worker; however, instead of being experienced simply as concern, it is experienced by the social worker as a persecutory anguish – so much so that it is unbearable and the social worker must flee.

Looking at this experience in relation to the schizophrenic client himself, we see that he cannot bear too much involvement from any source. He is, and seems to wish to be, isolated. He wanders alone with no intimate friends; he frequently misses social work appointments. One view of self-inflicted isolation is as a defence against being invaded and overwhelmed by such feelings as the social worker experienced. Paradoxically, however, and tragically, such isolation is recognised as psychic pain by the schizophrenic's mother and causes her increased anguish and worry, thus causing a vicious cycle of worry, withdrawal and increased worry. It could even be added that the schizophrenic cannot totally evade such feelings. They often manifest themselves in haunting and persecutory delusions that make the schizophrenic firmly believe that the world is plainly out to invade, or even kill, him.

Violence and projective identification

Violence proves to be another area where projective identification is carried out. The client who feels filled with inarticulate rage may crash into a social work office waving a knife or the approved social worker may be called to a situation where a person is 'out of control' waving knives and shouting abuse. The perfectly natural reaction is to feel fear, then the need for self-defence. We can act on each of these. We can run, or we can stand and fight. What may be being acted out, however, is a drama which originates within the client's own psyche. Thus if we feel fear, we may be being invaded by the frightened part of the client. The client is afraid of his or her own feelings – feelings which are so powerful that they seem to be violent. The consequent sense of panic is projected into others, including ourselves. We then, in our turn, become afraid and our judgement is clouded, leaving us liable to panic. It is at times such as this when our greatest asset is the ability to stay calm: to sit down when the client is standing up, speak quietly where the client is shouting, not do very much where the client is expecting a war. Our ability not to panic, to contain and provide a limit to the client's sense of being out of control may be the reason why he or she has come to us.

Having said this, the difficult balance to maintain, with regard to violence, is the need to escalate a situation as against the need to protect oneself. The prime motive must always be to care for oneself and, if we feel filled with dreadful and overpowering fear, then we are probably in a situation that is too much for us to handle. We should then have no qualms about either getting out of it – by running – or obtaining help as quickly as we safely can.

Projective identification and organisations

Projective identification can also be found operating between clients and organisations, within organisations, and between one organisation and another. An example would be the client who goes from one social work agency to another, using different names, cross-referencing problems or criticising other workers in their absence. A complex chain of intra-agency knots can be tied. These will defeat the agencies concerned, but also confirm the client's own negative self-image. The client has put into the respective agencies parts of him or herself, so that the agencies and their social workers act out the conflicts that the client normally feels internally. This can give the client some relief from the demands of his or her illness.

Social work and projective identification

The importance of the concept of projective identification for social workers is threefold.

First, if the unconscious motivation for projective identification is to control and distance the other person, then being aware of the process may act as a defence against being manipulated into acting against one's judgement or inclination. This is often the situation that social workers find that they are put into by both their clients and other agencies.

We should keep in mind the fact that in any situation, but especially ones where the protagonists have a strong emotional investment, there will be strong unconscious forces at work – forces which, by definition, we may know nothing about. Then we, at least, may be on our guard, and can aim to know our own minds.

This leads on to the second importance of the concept, which is to help us understand what, on the surface, will certainly seem to be very complex and mysterious events. This may not help us change these events, however. The events will have a life of their own and we as social workers will be coming on to the scene very late in the day. But understanding our own predicament when faced with these baffling events may give us clues as to what, at least, we ought not to do.

We may be talking about what seems to be an impossible task. Being aware of projective identification does not imply a sense of omniscience in the social worker – far from it. When we experience a sense of omniscience, we are more than likely to be in a process whereby the client, or his or her situation, has entered into us in such a way as to put into us all the possible feelings of goodness and benevolence which he or she finds too powerfully over-whelming to bear. The client feels small, inadequate and ignorant. We are the ones with insight and knowledge.

Thus, we can see that being aware of the process of projective identification implies far more than a desire for omniscience: it implies a readiness to accept the mystery of a situation and a client, and to let these become part of oneself. Listening to and feeling the responses in oneself then gives us a message as to what the client is experiencing.

A third aspect of projective identification for social workers thus emerges in the way in which it ascribes to us the role of caretaker for the most damaged, or damaging, aspects of our clients. We carry for our clients their despair, their failure, their anger – and sometimes their goodness and their achieve-ments. If we can contain these feelings and gradually, through the mediation of effective counselling and casework, hand them back in a non-punitive but accepting way, then we will be able to help our clients come to some clearer understanding of themselves and their predicaments. By helping them to integrate these unacknowledged and unwanted parts of their selves, we may help our clients gain more in integrity, self-respect and power.

Projective identification, therefore, carries a resource for us as social workers. It can make sense of some of the baffling and despairing situations that we encounter and which, no matter what we do, 'get inside us'. It can help us keep our feet on the ground when all about us are losing their heads and, more often than not, blaming it on us. It can help us to help the clients make more sense of their lives and themselves.

It does carry with it a price, however, which is that, to make full use of our feelings and intuition, we must become and remain open and sensitive to ourselves. This can be seen conversely in the situation where, because of a blind spot in ourselves, we continually encounter the same difficulty repeated in the lives of our clients; or in a similar way we, unconsciously, are drawn to those clients who most nearly represent our own internal needs.

Examples of this could be the social worker who repeatedly experiences violence in the course of his or her work; the social worker who often finds himself falling in love with his or her clients; the social worker who cannot say 'no'; the social worker who says 'no' too readily; the social worker whose clients are always teetering on the brink of breakdown (and need their social worker to keep them there).

If the client projectively identifies into us, we may, in our turn, projectively identify into the client. This can create difficulties for the progress of our work, unless properly understood and dealt with by the social worker through whatever means he or she finds most helpful. These can be many and various, but can range from supervision, to teamwork, to consultation, and perhaps, to psychotherapy or analysis for him or herself.

Impossible clients – impossible social work?

There is a tendency to consider the task and nature of social work in the effectiveness – or otherwise – of social workers' achievements in facilitating positive change (Payne, 1991; Rojek *et al.*, 1988; Davies, 1994; Reder *et al.*, 1993). This may be becoming a necessity, as we increasingly move into systems of performance monitoring and appraisal, on the one hand, and service specifications and unit costs on the other (Carter *et al.*, 1995). One method of defining the boundaries of social work action is through legislation and statutory instruments pertaining to the social work role (Davies, 1994). This can be amplified by considering the variety of roles or settings in which social workers function (Philpot and Hanvey, 1993). As Philpot and Hanvey, together with Pietroni (1995) observe, the very term social work 'is increasingly left out of policy and advisory guidance relating to community care' (Pietroni, 1995: 46).

One pertinent question is therefore: 'Is there a special role which social work embodies, and if so, how could this be illustrated?' Put another way, what is a social worker doing when he or she seems to be least effective?

We are not referring here to errors or judgements, mistakes, lapses or even deliberate case of malpractice, but to quite the opposite: to the nature of social work which enables or requires a social worker to work with clients year in, year out, sometimes with some clients that other services do not want to know, who might have even received the label of being impossible.

By 'impossible' is meant those clients on our caseload whom we feel unable to help. This may be a rather unpopular concept at present. Local authorities are increasingly, and appropriately, called to account through such measures as the Citizens' Charter and the Data Protection and Freedom of Information Acts. Individual social work practice is now subject to close scrutiny as, for instance, in the mental health review tribunal system for compulsory detained psychiatric patients. Taken together with user participation in service provision, and the drive towards empowerment, we are experiencing – theoretically at any rate – a potential for greater democratisation of services against authoritarianism and the 'disabling professions' (Illich, 1977). These measures may also be attempts to provide a legitimation for an undermining of social workers' morale.

Nevertheless, we do encounter service users and clients who present us individually with difficulties in helping. Sometimes, these problems ripple out, to cause our organisations problems too – occasionally with individual social workers themselves as the focus of the 'problem'.

Taking account of our statutory responsibilities to remain involved with people who might not want our assistance, how can we remain involved in a helpful way? 'Impossible' clients are, in the definition referred to here, clients who put themselves outside the range of most agencies, whether therapeutic or punitive. Generally, this group of service users might commit petty crime, but nothing sufficiently serious to warrant custodial sentences or probation. They might use alcohol or drugs in destructive ways. They might harm themselves and need occasional short hospital admissions to recover, but quickly discharge themselves, yet present as insufficiently 'at risk' to need compulsory detention under the Mental Health Act. They might have children on an 'at risk' register, yet hover on the borders of concern, retaining charge of their children despite concerns about parenting. They might display antisocial behaviour, or assault people or professionals, but in minor ways, and so avoid custodial sentence or psychiatric assessment. Such clients may even be barred from social service offices due to 'disruptive behaviour'.

Barring clients from social services, or denying access to services can be ways of punishing people for what might be classified as undesirable behaviour. This may be even more of a temptation in relation to community care legislation, where access to services depends on an assessment of need. One trigger factor may be demonstration of commitment which might be lacking in service users who are, for whatever reason, difficult to engage with.

Psychiatry has rationalised these dilemmas in a descriptive way by invoking the diagnosis of 'personality disorder'. The definition of personality disorder according to the International Classification of Diseases (ICD-10), which is a definition adopted by the World Health Organisation is as follows:

> Deeply ingrained maladaptive patterns of behaviour generally recognisable by the time of adolescence or earlier and continuing throughout most of adult life, although often becoming less obvious in middle age. The personality is abnormal either in the balance of its components, their quality and expression or in its total aspect. As a result either the patient or society suffers or both. (Wolf *et al.*, 1990)

There are several varieties of personality disorder in psychiatric diagnosis. These include the paranoid, the schizoid, the hysterical, the obsessional, the affective, the narcissistic and the inadequate personality. In relation to a discussion about the 'impossible client', the manifestation of what is termed the 'borderline personality disorder' is probably of most relevance. This is a complicated term, introduced from psychoanalysis in the USA (Kernberg, 1975, 1993), and refers essentially to clients who are neither psychotic, nor neurotic, but who experience profound problems in making and sustaining relationships, resorting in times of stress or crisis to self-harm or destructive acts.

Psychiatry is a controversial area for social workers, who often turn to social theorists, or models based on positions opposed to traditional psychiatry such as the radical 'anti-psychiatry' movement for alternative constructions or explanations of distress. These perspectives may see 'insanity' as a sane response to an insane world. Bateson (1973), and Laing (1975), are two of the key originators of such ideas as the 'double-bind' in the explanation of psychosis. Breggin (1993) draws together a number of viewpoints and testimonies – some from survivors of the psychiatric system. Nevertheless psychotic clients continue to be arrested or 'sectioned', or both. Indeed, it is the statutory duty of an approved social worker to make an application for hospital admission if he or she feels that this is appropriate (Mental Health Act 1983, section 13 (1)).

However, the diagnosis of 'personality disorder' is not, by itself, a reason to detain someone under the Mental Health Act. A person with a suspected diagnosis of personality disorder could, if in need of an assessment and if it were justified in the interests of their health and safety or that of others, be so admitted as an emergency under section 4 or for 28 days under section 2. However, for a longer period of treatment, say under sections 3 or 37, he or she would have to be regarded as being treatable (Jones, 1994). More often, the diagnosis of personality disorder can be used as an exclusion clause on the part of doctors and social workers to avoid having to try to hospitalise and treat such a patient. Correspondingly, many of our clients will not have come into contact with psychiatric services nor engendered a 'diagnosis' of any disorder. Here we focus on those of our clients who experience distress in organisations, whilst appearing to evoke helplessness or even dislike amongst those who have the task of helping.

Case example 2: Alf

Alf was a young man in his early twenties at the first point of referral. He lived at home with his parents and had had a number of short admissions to psychiatric hospital, usually following transfer from prison for minor offences, such as trying car door handles. Following his first referral to social services, he was ascribed a diagnosis of schizophrenia. The referral came to the approved social worker for assistance with leaving hospital and going home.

Assistance was given in the form of supportive counselling with Alf individually and with his mother and father. Alf's mother appeared to be extremely anxious about her son's welfare. Alf's father seemed rather remote and to adopt rather cool attitudes about his son's 'bad behaviour'. Alf returned home, and the approved social worker continued to visit to offer support and monitoring in the event of Alf relapsing. As the approved social worker got to know Alf better, the frightening world he inhabited was revealed.

Alf felt, quite concretely, that he was in great danger from sources outside his home, and indeed revealed that, for many years, he had slept with a knife under his pillow. It was agreed that it might be best for Alf if he were to work towards leaving home by first living more independently with continuing support. This was achieved, and Alf was established in council bedsitting accommodation. Shortly after this, his parents left the city and moved many miles away. Gradually, Alf's mental state seemed to improve. He felt less paranoid, and displayed no criminal behaviour. Then, due to the vicissitudes of social service caseload priorities, the approved social worker was forced to close Alf as an active case.

Some months later, Alf was referred, using drugs. He was not admitted to psychiatric hospital, or an addiction clinic because he did not appear to be an 'addict'. He was ascribed the diagnosis of personality disorder. As acting team manager, the approved social worker resumed the support which he had previously been offering him – regular visits, befriending, advising on practical matters, welfare rights and so on. Alf seemed to respond to this. He began to reorganise his life, and the offending behaviour did not recur.

Contact with Alf slipped once more, because administrative priorities began to present themselves, and the view was taken that he was becoming independent. Visits diminished. Several months passed by, until one day he presented himself in the office. He looked dishevelled and dirty, with long, unkempt hair. His clothes were smelly and his nails dirty. He said he had got into drugs in a big way. He was frightened, because people had taken over his flat, and were not allowing him back in. He had been arrested for possession of drugs, but released on bail.

The approved social worker agreed to help. He visited Alf's flat and found that it had been taken over by some difficult individuals. With the assistance of the housing department and the police, removal was effected. By this time, Alf was too frightened to return there. The hospital would not admit him because he was not 'mentally ill' (his most recent diagnosis being personality disorder), so an emergency placement was found in a night shelter, followed by a transfer to some homeless persons accommodation. Eventually, Alf was rehoused, and was allocated to another social worker who ensured continuing support and the adoption of a no-closure policy in this particular case. Subsequently, Alf remained out of trouble and avoided institutional confinement.

Comment

This example illustrates some of the difficulties faced by a practitioner attempting to work in a way dedicated to continuing care, against the priorities of increasingly reduced statutory priorities. Alf appeared to find value in the maintenance of a social work relationship, although this could only accurately be perceived in the way in which he began to fall apart when the safety net of the relationship dissipated. In the face of consistent and overwhelming priorities it is difficult to retain a sense of the importance of sustaining a long-term relationship with a client where nothing is going wrong.

Case example 3: Brenda

Brenda had been admitted to psychiatric hospital in her adolescence, following disturbed behaviour at home – hitting strangers in the street and exposing herself in a sexually disinhibited manner. It emerged, through assessments, that she was the victim of sexual and physical abuse. The perpetrator – her father – disappeared from the scene and, gradually, Brenda's disturbances eased. However, she continued to refer herself, or be referred, to the local outpatient clinic, either for psychiatric or medical assessment. In her early adulthood, she had become a parent herself, but her children spent most of their time with her mother.

Like Alf, Brenda had moved from an early diagnosis of schizophrenia, to a later diagnosis of personality disorder. At the many referrals, psychiatrists tended to be reluctant to admit Brenda to hospital on the basis of the later diagnosis, whilst the approved social workers tended to accept the spirited and well argued defence against admission put up by Brenda's family. Consequently, hospital admission was never effected. However, and somewhat paradoxically, due to staffing constraints in the local social services office, Brenda was never allocated a social worker because of the absence of positive risk to herself or others.

A crisis occurred one weekend when Brenda turned up in a local cafe, partly clothed, and talking incoherently. The cafe owner contacted the police for assistance, who referred the matter to the emergency duty social worker. She discussed with the police the possibility of using section 136 to remove Brenda to a 'place of safety', but the police inspector declined on the basis that a cafe was not clearly a place of business. Although this was clearly debatable, the important factor in the social worker's mind was to ensure that Brenda received help. She therefore contacted a section 12 approved doctor, and succeeded in admitting Brenda to hospital under an emergency power of the Mental Health Act, section 4. When the duty senior registrar examined her the following morning, it was found that Brenda was displaying no positive symptoms of mental illness, and that the section order should not be allowed to continue beyond the 72 hours of its duration. The following day, Brenda discharged herself from hospital and visited the social services area office. On being asked to wait to see a duty social worker, she shouted and became so disruptive that she had to be escorted from the building.

Comment

The example of Brenda not only highlights how despair and fragmentation can be perpetuated through generations but also demonstrates the ways in which the effects of sexual abuse can manifest themselves through mental illness. Resource constraints in the local social services offices contributed to the sense of continuous crisis in Brenda's life and that of her children and family. Two issues were involved: the problem of separating adult services from children's services and the problems that can arise between professional teams working within the same agency, as well as between agencies. For example, the emergency duty social worker felt that the area office was neglecting Brenda, but the area office was bound by overwhelming pressures of crises on duty and therefore felt unable to allocate Brenda.

Relations between the emergency duty team and the police became rather strained over the interpretation of section 136. Relations between social services and the hospital were frayed as a result of what was perceived as a peremptory discharge arrangement. In the middle of all this, Brenda was in some kind of distress, yet had become removed from all available services.

Commentary

In a volume of Winnicott's collected papers, *The Maturational Processes and the Facilitating Environment* (1963), a paper entitled 'The Psychotherapy of the Character Disorders' is followed by one entitled 'The Mentally Ill in Your Caseload', delivered by Winnicott to the then Association of Social Workers in 1963. Taken together, these two papers provide some crucial insights into social work with people who seem to present unresolvable difficulties. In the former paper, Winnicott highlights, amongst other things, the part society plays in accepting or creating difficulties for such individuals (ibid.: 205). In the latter paper, he provides some discussion of the social work role. One key quotation he employs is from another psychoanalyst, Rickman: 'Mental illness consists in not being able to find anyone who can stand you' (ibid.: 218).

In the illustrations cited above and in others of the author's experience, the social work role consisted of providing a presence that could withstand some of the difficulties encountered by – and, indeed, occasionally presented by – the client. These are areas in which we feel uneasy. To acknowledge that we find any of our clients 'impossible' may be unpalatable. Yet individual social workers and organisational systems do turn against clients, as I have tried to demonstrate above, and often with very reasoned, even libertarian arguments (for example, 'health and safety' in the case of a 'dangerous' client).

Another of Winnicott's themes is the way that hatred must be acknowledged, and worked through, so that a position of hope can be arrived at (Winnicott, 1947). This brings us back to social work morale. Social workers often feel hated, and are made to feel unwanted, either individually by some of their clients, publicly by the media, or implicitly in the struggle for the recognition of the social work role in debates about public policy. For example it could be interpreted that the impulse to abolish the mental hospitals has represented the wish to abolish the despair of mental illness. The ability to tolerate despair and help each other survive it might be a communal task which social work as a profession needs to recognise in order not only to survive, but to flourish.

11 Ethical issues in approved social work

Introduction

This chapter reviews the approved social worker's role in sections 115, 137, 138, 29 and 135 of the Mental Health Act 1983, which form boundaries of the approved social worker's role. This role can result in stressful decisions involving professional and personal ethics, with additional implications for health, safety and good practice.

The role of the approved social worker was established in the Mental Health Act 1983 (Prior, 1992). Approved social workers are qualified social workers who have had two years' post-qualification experience before becoming eligible for approved social work training (Huxley, 1993). Approved social work training consists of a 60-day training programme provided by local authorities and approved by the CCETSW. Only social services authorities have the power to appoint approved social workers, (Jones, 1996). On completion of their training programme, approved social workers are assessed in relation to 39 competence and performance criteria (CCETSW paper 19.19). As a result of their training and experience, they are expected to have specialist knowledge of mental disorder (Hoggett, 1996) and it is their duty to make an application for admission to hospital or guardianship where they are satisfied that it ought to be made and that there are no suitable alternatives to admission (Mental Health Act, section 13 (1)).

This chapter explores some implications for the approved social worker in relation to professional and personal ethics. In this regard, it is important to note that, when carrying out duties under section 13, the approved social worker holds a personal liability for their actions (Jones, 1996).

Literature review

Michael Sheppard (1990) examined the approved social worker's role in assessment, and developed a standardised assessment schedule. Subsequently, Sheppard elucidated some of the complexities of the approved social worker's decision-making role, highlighting the need to take account of cultural factors, racism, sexism, as well as the capacity to use a wide variety of professional skills (Sheppard, 1991). Dave Sheppard (1991) observes that the approved social worker needs to take into account 11 factors before making any decision. The development of the approved social worker's role in practice, including some of the subsequent contradictions and complications of that role, has increasingly been recognised (Prior, 1992; Barnes *et al.*, 1990; Huxley and Kerfoot, 1994). The relationship between the notion of an ethical base for approved social workers and the core value base as defined by the CCETSW has perhaps remained rather more dormant. Professional ethics are not mentioned explicitly in CCETSW's paper 19.19, although seven core values are identified (p.25). O'Hagan (1986, 1994) has critically discussed the lack of an ethical foundation in writings on crisis intervention.

The Mental Health Act Commission, commenting on their consultation with approved social workers, report that their role should be wider than merely responding to crisis requests for admission, yet, at the same time, the approved social worker's role seems to have become constricted by increasing emphases on 'completing forms' and 'statutory duties' (Mental Health Act Commission, 1995). Mayberry (1996) has undertaken work on ethical issues surrounding the removal of patients from home under section 47 of the National Assistance Act 1948. Atkinson (1996) considers some problems posed by the Mental Health (Patients in the Community) Act 1995 and community supervision registers in relation to social control. This chapter will focus on social work aspects of the Mental Health Act 1983.

Practice discussions

There are sections of the Act which can place approved social workers in an invidious and precarious position with regard to their professional duties and individual responsibility – a position which evokes dilemmas touching on professional and personal ethics. These are especially evident in circumstances where an approved social worker is suddenly, and sometimes unexpectedly, confronted with a decision which only he or she is empowered to make (unlike, say, the more frequently cited sections 2, 3, 4, 7, or 136, where either doctors or police officers will also necessarily be involved). In that sense, such circumstances are referred to in this chapter as being on the outer limits of the approved social worker's responsibilities and duties.

Confirmation of that location might be found in the *Statistical Bulletin* issued by the Department of Health in 1996, which has a record of inpatient figures for people formally detained under the Mental Health Act 1983. It contains no record for the following sections of the Act:

- Section 115: the approved social worker's power to inspect a premises in which a mentally ill person might be living
- Section 129: making it an offence to obstruct an approved social worker in the performance of his or her duties
- Sections 137–138: the approved social worker's power to retake a patient who is escaping during an assessment
- Section 29: the powers of a county court on the application of an approved social worker to appoint a nearest relative.

These sections shall now be discussed in more detail, making use of relevant case material.

Section 115

An Approved Social Worker ... may ... enter and inspect any premises ... in which a mentally disordered person is living, if he has reasonable cause to believe that the patient is not under proper care. (Mental Health Act, section 115)

As Jones (1996) points out, this is not a power to force access and, if forced access is required, recourse should be made to section 135 provisions. However in the experience of the author, most people do not refuse access if proper and careful explanation of the circumstances is offered. Two examples illustrate circumstances in which power of entry was needed.

Case examples

A man was admitted to psychiatric hospital in a catatonic and mute state. It was not possible to elicit any agreement or disagreement from this man to check whether his flat was properly secured, the gas switched off and so on. On these grounds, the approved social worker involved invoked his powers under section 115 to open the door of the man's flat, verify that all was safe and sound – including that there were no pets left unattended – and then ensured the flat was left secure.

In the second case, an approved social worker and GP visited a man about whom the GP was concerned. The man was not at home, but his door was ajar. The approved social worker took the view that section 115 powers permitted entry in the absence of the tenant (the GP's patient) in order to check whether the man was at home, and to assess the situation. The patient was not at home, but his flat was in a state of extreme disorder, indicating that perhaps he had left abruptly and was in need of some further assistance.

Comment

Although in each of these examples the approved social worker felt a personal disinclination to trespass onto a person's private residence, the statutory duty to ensure protection of property and/or to carry out an appropriate assessment overrode personal inclination.

Section 129

> ... Any person who ... obstructs ... [an ASW] ... in the exercise of his functions shall be guilty of an offence. (Mental Health Act 1983 [MHA], quoted in Jones, 1996, p. 336)

Jones (1996) links this with section 115, indicating that one possible course of action, should entry be refused, would be for the approved social worker to cite section 129 as such a refusal is an offence. This is certainly a possible approach, although in some situations it might escalate an atmosphere of already heightened tension. The danger of using this approach without regard to the distress it may cause was demonstrated in the following case example.

Case example

A woman living alone opened her door slightly to the assessment team of two doctors and approved social worker. On discovering their reason for being there, she did not speak, but did not allow anyone to enter her flat either.

The approved social worker attempted to persuade her to allow the assessment team into her flat in order to check that she was caring for herself adequately and, in so doing, mentioned the possibility of an offence being committed under section 129 if access was refused. This achieved the opposite of the desired effect. This client's paranoid state of mind was such that she immediately closed the door on the assessment team.

The threat of the sanction of section 129 in discussions with a local family health services authority who refused to divulge the name of a patient's GP did succeed in obtaining a swift and positive agreement to release that piece of information. Using this same tactic in negotiations with a police officer who was unable to send officers to assist an approved social worker in a potentially dangerous assessment led to an amicable discussion with that officer's supervisor, who agreed to have a constable on 'standby'.

Comment

Whilst it may be useful to have in reserve the legal sanctions of section 129 in cases of extreme resistance, such measures need to be used sensitively and with specific regard to the exigencies of each situation.

Sections 137–138

Section 137 (1) creates a situation where a person being conveyed or detained as a result of a mental health assessment is in legal custody, whilst section 137 (2) confers on an approved social worker the powers of a police constable. Section 138 empowers a police constable or approved social worker to retake any such person who might be escaping (or has previously escaped, subject to certain time restrictions). Linking these powers with the approved social worker's personal liability for their actions, there can arise a situation where an approved social worker is in the difficult position of recognising that someone needs to be restrained from fleeing, having a legal power to restrain them, but in the absence of adequate back up – either from police, departmental colleagues or ambulance crew – needs to allow the patient to go or risk physical harm to themselves. Provided the approved social worker can be shown to have acted 'in good faith' and to the best of their ability and judgement at the time, it is unlikely that they could be held culpable in such a situation. The 'duty of care' in health and safety legislation applies as much to the preservation of one's own life as to the lives of others.

Case examples

A female client was assessed by an approved social worker and two doctors, who agreed that the client needed to be admitted to hospital. The doctors were unable to stay, and the police and ambulance crews had not arrived by the agreed appointed time.

The client proceeded to flee the family home where the assessment had taken place. The family members were too distressed to try to restrain her, but insisted that she was an active suicide risk. The approved social worker therefore followed at a discreet distance. By chance, a police van drew up at traffic lights as the client was crossing the road, and the officers present agreed to assist the approved social worker in escorting the client to hospital.

In another case, the approved social worker, fearing for the safety of the client and himself, restrained the client by holding his wrists until the police arrived.

Comment

These instances highlight in particular the problem of how far an approved social worker might need to go in order to feel that they have acted 'in good faith' to fulfil their statutory duties. Placing oneself in excessive danger could, arguably, not be acting with reasonable care towards one's own safety as is required by health and safety legislation.

Section 29

> The county court may ... direct ... that the functions of the nearest relative ... be exercisable by the applicant (who may be an Approved Social Worker). (MHA, quoted in Jones, 1996, p.147)

The Mental Health Act confers specific and important powers on a client's 'nearest relative', and there is a strict hierarchy of who is or can be, a person's nearest relative (ibid., 29). Section 29 creates the possibility of varying that hierarchy, on application to a county court, in circumstances where:

a) a person has no nearest relative within the meaning of the Act – or it is not reasonably practicable to ascertain whether such a one exists or not;
b) the nearest relative is incapable of acting as such by reason of mental disorder or other illness;
c) the nearest relative unreasonably objects to the making of an application for treatment or guardianship;
d) the nearest relative has exercised without due regard to the welfare of the patient or the interests of the public his power to discharge the patient from hospital or guardianship. (MHA, quoted in Jones, 1996, p.147)

Clearly this is a power which an approved social worker must use with caution. Local authorities may themselves be unwilling to assume the powers of an 'acting nearest relative' partly because of the ethical nature of displacing a person's next of kin in favour of a local authority officer, but also because of the consequent time and resources which become committed to that individual (Hoggett, 1996).

The following two examples focus on cases in which section 29 was invoked because of an assessment made by the approved social worker based on clause (c) above – that, in each case, the formal nearest relative was felt to be acting 'unreasonably' in withholding consent for treatment to proceed. Hoggett poses the question 'will it ever be reasonable for the relative to disagree with professional opinions?' (Hoggett, 1996: 61), but goes on to illustrate an instance where a county court judge had indeed declined to find that the nearest relative was acting unreasonably because the patient's detention was no longer deemed to be necessary for the protection of other persons.

Case examples

In the first example, an elderly person had become depressed to the point of refusing food and liquid, refusing medication and becoming electively mute. The responsible medical officer and GP decided that ECT was required to save her life. The client's family, however, felt that this woman had enjoyed a long and active life and would not wish to have her life prolonged by ECT. The approved social worker decided that the family was acting unreasonably. He asked the social services' legal department to proceed with a section 29 application so that treatment could be given.

The second example concerns a young man who had committed a serious criminal offence and appeared to be suffering from a mental illness. Having been detained in a police station, he was admitted to hospital for assessment at the instigation of the arresting officer. The doctors recommended treatment but his nearest relative objected. Given the risk to the safety of others, as well as concerns over the patient's own health and safety, the approved social worker felt that this objection was unreasonable, and made application for the displacement of the nearest relative.

Comment

These examples highlight the approved social worker's need to avoid becoming a 'psy-expert' (Howe, 1996), or 'secular priest' (North, 1972) in trying to enforce conformity on clients and their families. Issues of when and how far to intervene are at the heart of the approved social worker's ethical practice. Again, perhaps, we are reminded of the caution expressed by Prior (1992) and Atkinson (1996) about the uses and potential abuses of power in contemporary mental health policy: 'Order (law) is preferred to freedom, to the extent of that the abuses of order (law) will be preferred to the abuses of freedom' (Atkinson, 1996: 123).

In the meantime, the tension for approved social workers is to continue to provide a mental health service, as arbiters of these complex and uneasy dilemmas.

Conclusions

The sections referred to – 115, 129, 137, 138, 29 – encompass a range of ethical and practice issues which can confront an approved social worker. It is relatively rare for these sections to be invoked and, when they are, it can involve tensions and stress for the worker. The case studies presented in this chapter suggest the following guidelines for practice:

1   There is a need for approved social workers to be clear about their own personal value bases – for example, when to forcibly intervene in a client's life, issues of self-determination and empowerment as against issues of personal and public safety. Deliberations on these issues must always be grounded in clinical and legal knowledge.
2   There is a need to ensure that health and safety requirements are observed with due regard to 'duty of care' to self as well as others. There is also a need to pay attention to the lessons of public inquiries and past incidents. Rojek *et al.*, in their discussion of the murder of social workers, state: 'the depiction of the social as an environment of cosy, relaxed and secure intimacy is misleading' (Rojek *et al.*, 1988: 152).
3   There is a need to have good working relationships with the police, ambulance service and legal colleagues in order to be able to support one another in carrying out difficult and stressful duties. The members of the multidisciplinary assessment team need to work together cohesively.
4   There is a need for adequate organisation and management of approved social workers' services, including support and supervision by managers experienced in approved social work. Local authorities are now required to provide a programme of regular refresher training to approved social workers (CCETSW, 1994).

Section 135: the legal framework

The Mental Health Act 1983 gives its section 135 the heading 'Warrant to search for and remove patients' (MHA quoted in Jones, 1996, p.349). The provisions of this section enable an approved social worker to apply to a magistrate for a warrant to empower a constable to enter, by force if necessary, a premises where the approved social worker has 'reasonable cause' to suspect a mentally disordered person:

a) has been, or is being, ill-treated, neglected, or kept otherwise than under proper control, in any place within the jurisdiction of the justices, or

b) being unable to care for himself is living alone in any such place. (Jones, 1996: 238–9)

Although the warrant is directed to a police constable, the constable must be accompanied by an approved social worker and a doctor (a 'registered medical practitioner' in terms of the Act) who may, or may not be, a psychiatrist.

Section 135 allows entry, by force if need be, and removal to a 'place of safety' (Jones, 1994: 239) for up to 72 hours in order that a full assessment within the terms of the Act can take place. However, in view of the rights of patients to a full and early assessment, it is generally accepted as good practice amongst approved social workers to make that assessment at the point of entry to a person's premises, rather than convey him or her elsewhere.

The approved social worker need not be convinced that a person is mentally ill in order to apply for a section 135 warrant but, rather, needs to demonstrate 'reasonable cause' to suspect that an assessment is necessary, on the grounds outlined above. In other words, it is possible to force access to a person's home and not subsequently remove them to hospital; conversely, it may not be necessary to use section 135 to force access if, on arrival at a person's home, the approved social worker has good reason not to authorise forced entry.

It is important to consider section 135 in the context of two other sections of the Act. The first is section 13 (1), which creates a mandatory duty laid upon the approved social worker to make an application under the Act if he or she believes an application ought to be made (Jones, 1994: 50). In other words, an approved social worker cannot evade the requirement to go through the process of an assessment and application, even it if involves the tortuous and arguably anti-libertarian strictures of section 135, in order to meet their obligations under section 13 (1). Furthermore, this obligation is a personal one, in that the approved social worker, when implementing the Act, is meant to exercise their own judgement and not act at the behest of the employer: The independence of the approved social worker's judgement is meant to be near to sacrosanct and this point is heavily emphasised in approved social work training. Nevertheless, this still appears to be not always comprehended or understood by psychiatrists or GPs, who still tend to regard the approved social worker as peripheral, rather than central, to the process of deciding about compulsory admission. This can also perhaps be seen reflected in the one small chapter (six pages out of 717 in total) dedicated to the role of the 'hospital social worker' in the 1991 edition of the UCH *Textbook of Psychiatry* (Wolff *et al.*, 1991) – although conversely, it could be said, positively, that social work is at least mentioned in a textbook on psychiatry!

Numbers involved

The DoH *Statistical Bulletin 1996/10* gives the following figures for section 135 applications for England and Wales:

*   1989–90:   87
*   1990–91:   81
*   1991–92:   99
*   1992–93:   128
*   1993–94:   108
*   1994–95:   145

The general increase in the numbers of applications reflects a general increase in the use of formal admissions. The most recent full-year statistic available from the city district from where the case example 'Sam' (page 172) derives is 12 incidents of section 135 warrants being requested (out of an overall population of around 230 000 people), of which three incidents were for the same person, who succeeded in either avoiding assessment (in the case of the first application) or of returning home whilst confined to hospital under section, necessitating approved social work involvement in forcing entry to her home to ensure her return (in the case of the two subsequent applications). Of those 12 applications the race and gender breakdown was as follows:

*   White males: 3 (including two separate applications for one individual)
*   White females: 7 (including three separate applications for one individual)
*   Black males: 1
*   Black females: 1

The process of application

An application for a section 135 warrant is made to a magistrates' court by an approved social worker. Outside court hours, arrangements should be made locally to have access to a magistrates' rota, possibly through local police stations. However, for emergency access to property – for example in order to guarantee immediate life and limb protection, or where a constable is 'in pursuit' of a fugitive – no warrant may be necessary, although this will be a matter to be judged in individual cases. (Jones (1994) provides a fuller account of common law provisions and the ways in which the Police and Criminal Evidence Act of 1984 affects such circumstances.)

An application involves the approved social worker visiting the court, and presenting two pieces of paper, the first being a 'statement of facts' about the case, explaining why a warrant is felt necessary. The court keeps this, as their evidence. The second paper is the warrant itself, which is signed by the magistrate and which the approved social worker retains as his or her evidence to bring before the police in order to enlist their services in assisting in its execution.

The police and ambulance services will then be coordinated, bringing them together at the same time as the doctor (or, ideally, two doctors) if a full and complete mental health assessment is to take place. Correspondingly, the local hospital service will need to be alerted to begin the process of finding a bed.

The organisation of a section 135 assessment requires quite considerable organisational skills, together with fine professional judgements, such as whether the approved social worker routinely have police, or ambulance, or doctors present. It may be preferable, in terms of sensitive and anti-oppressive practice, to start off with the approved social worker. However, given the need to observe health and safety requirements, this may be too minimal a presence, and at least one other colleague ought to be present. Tragically, at least one approved social worker – Norma Morris of the London Borough of Haringey in 1987 – has been murdered in the attempted performance of her duties, when left alone with a psychotic client. It is the view of the author that it ought to be mandatory advice for approved social workers never to be in the position of being alone with a client subject to a formal assessment. This is implied, although not clearly stated, in the Mental Health Act Commission Code of Practice (section 11).

It may be that the client has already given sufficient indications that entry for assessment will be refused. Informal visits may well have already been unsuccessfully attempted. Certainly, unless in the case of immediate emergency, good practice would indicate that informal attempts to engage clients in receiving voluntary help ought to be made prior to a formal mental health assessment. There begins to emerge, therefore, an incremental judgement about the minimum amount of intrusive presence necessary in order to ensure an adequate and safe assessment.

Further complicating factors which arise are the logistics about the availability of police personnel to guarantee the safety of all involved, the availability of ambulances and the availability of hospital beds. For example, it will not be possible, or safe, to contain or restrain a disturbed client for a long period while hospital managers and nursing managers argue about the availability of a bed. It may be better to clarify the position about bed availability before an assessment proceeds. In the experience of the author this can lead to approved social workers refusing to conduct an assessment unless a bed is identified in advance, thereby placing themselves conceivably in conflict with section 13 (1) (the 'personal liability' clause) for which they might need union assistance if management is not sufficiently aware of the tensions and safety problems associated with forced access, forced assessment and forced removal of people from their own homes – albeit, people with life-threatening illnesses.

Conveyance to hospital

It is the approved social worker's responsibility to ensure the safe arrival of the patient and the legal documents authorising detention (the 'section papers') at the hospital, at more or less the same time. The approved social worker is not advised to take the patient in their own transport – the guidance issued by the Mental Health Act Commission Code of Practice is that ambulance transport is the recommended means, in terms of anti-oppressive practice, civil rights and access to medical and nursing treatment whilst in transit (Mental Health Act Commission Code, in Jones, 1994: 442–3). Furthermore, in order for all professionals to feel that appropriate responsibility is being taken by the approved social worker, he or she should normally travel with the patient in the ambulance. Clearly, this too can then cause problems for the approved social worker in returning to their own car, in terms of practicability and in remote country districts or in terms of parking restrictions and 'tow-away zones' in cities. Too few local authorities seem to have any capacity for issuing approved social workers with parking waivers, despite the need for readily available transport.

Case example: Sam

Sam had been a general concern to her general practitioner and her neighbours for several weeks. She had been heard shouting and banging in her flat, and had stopped taking antipsychotic medication. Her GP had visited her and found her to be in a delusional state of mind, believing that the world was about to come to an end. As if to confirm Sam's paranoia, her children had been removed several months previously due to severe neglect.

Officers in the local social services' office appeared to be reluctant to agree with her general practitioner that this lady needed a mental health assessment. As days went by, the banging stopped and the client ceased answering the door to her GP. Due to staff shortages, the local office manager had not been able to allocate Sam a social worker of her own. Minor fires then began to break out in Sam's flat, causing consternation to her neighbours. The fire brigade had called and been able to douse the flames, but immediately Sam locked her doors and withdrew into herself.

An approved social worker from the newly formed mental health team was then contacted. He felt that a section 135 warrant was appropriate on the grounds that Sam was both living alone, and was being kept 'otherwise than under proper control'. He therefore made an application on both these grounds, although was advised by the magistrate that the second ground could only really apply if Sam had been living under someone else's care but was not kept 'under control'. Nevertheless, given the concern about Sam's risk to herself, through self-neglect, and to the public on a fairly large scale, through fire-raising, the magistrate left both grounds in the statement of facts and the warrant.

In organising access to the flat, the approved social worker needed all three emergency services – the police, to execute the warrant and for safety, the ambulance service for conveyance, and the fire brigade, to check for fire hazards and gain direct access through Sam's window, as the door was locked, bolted and reinforced. Sam offered no resistance to admission once access had been effected.

At the request of the approved social worker, her GP and a psychiatrist were both present. She was placed under section 3 of the Mental Health Act, empowering detention for up to six months for medical treatment. She made a good recovery in hospital, although she needed several months of inpatient treatment, followed by gradual and planned discharge.

Comment

The case of Sam illustrates some of the delicate legal judgements and interpretation involved in deciding upon a section 135. This example also illustrates the ways in which social factors (for example, the removal of Sam's child) combined with the inability of some services to either follow support through, or undertake preventive work, can lead to a situation which necessitates a compulsory admission which might otherwise have been avoided. Nevertheless, had the approved social worker failed to act when he did, Sam could have been placed at far more serious risk and might well have died and caused the death of others.

The events described in relation to Sam took place over a period of several months. During this time, the social services department involved was being restructured from a generic, patch-based service, into specialist, client-group services. It was an approved social worker from the new specialist mental health team who initiated the section 135 proceedings. It did not prove possible to review the local area decision not to pursue a full mental health assessment earlier, because most of the staff involved left during the months following what proved to be a somewhat acrimonious restructuring.

Had suitable mental health support and intervention been available at an earlier stage, a formal admission under the Mental Health Act might have been avoided or, if not avoided completely, the necessity for the full-scale intervention of all the emergency services (police, fire brigade and ambulance) might have been averted and a calmer admission been effected. As it was, allowing a situation to slip into an ever-deepening crisis created the need for drastic action.

These factors point to the desirability of social work staff both to be more attuned to mental health needs in general, as well as the necessity for the ready availability of advice and support to area teams from approved social workers as recommended in the Richie Report into the murder of Jonathan Zito by Christopher Clunis (Richie, 1994). They also point to the requirement to retain a need for client responsibility and client contact despite any reorganisations or restructuring undertaken by social service departments.

The negative impact of organisational factors and resource pressures on service users and practitioners is discussed in the *Woodley Team Report* (1995) following a homicide by a person suffering a severe mental illness. It might also be observed how crucial it is, therefore, to try to avoid interdepartmental acrimony and create proper staff support systems so that staff feel that their own anxieties are being managed. The impact of stress is increasingly being recognised by the social work media and, it is hoped, social service departments (*Community Care*, 9, 16 February 1996).

A final point to note is that Sam was a black woman. The delays in appropriate social work meant that Sam was at once denied a positive service (counselling, for example), whilst consequently subjected to forced intervention, which added to any sense she might have had of the persecutory and racist nature of the psychiatric services (Fernando, 1991, 1995). Racism, civil liberties and anti-oppressive practice need to be carefully considered in all aspects of social work, but especially in areas where such large-scale and personal authority is employed, as in the approved social worker's powers under the Mental Health Act. Conversely, services must not be denied to people because of their skin colour (as also highlighted in the Richie Report). This example illustrates how organisational problems can combine with misjudgements to create an oppressive system.

Ethical issues

Clearly it is a major step to force access into someone's private property. In order to have the authority to do this, the approved social worker must apply to a magistrate and offer sufficient evidence.

It is worthwhile noting that, under section 115 of the Mental Health Act, it is an offence to prohibit access to an approved social worker who may, at all reasonable times, be given access to 'enter and inspect' a property where he or she believes a mentally disordered person is living if he or she has reasonable cause to suspect that the patient is not receiving proper care, whilst section 129 makes it an offence to unreasonably obstruct an approved social worker in the performance of his or her duties. These latter powers are not, however, a power to force access where access is denied – to achieve that, in the absence of clear and urgent risk to life, section 135 needs to be invoked. For example, Jones (1994) offers the suggestion that, if entry under section 115 is refused, the approved social worker could point out that this refusal could constitute an offence under section 129, which exposition could impress the person refusing access sufficiently to cause them to open up and allow entry. If it did not achieve that end, access under section 135 could then be sought (Jones, 1994: 205). In the sense of offering the need for recourse to formal court proceedings, section 135 should act as a protection for patients/clients.

An approved social worker's refusal to consider section 135, whilst arguably not being lawful, could, as demonstrated above, result in a dangerous situation becoming more dangerous.

Conversely, the use of section 135 needs to be applied sensitively if approved social workers are not to be considered as monitors and arbiters of the freedom of thought. The debate about the overuse of psychiatric medication (see, for example, the letters page of the *Independent*, 19 June 1995), together with criticism from such clinicians as Breggin (1993) highlight these considerations which become more important in the context of the Mental Health (Patients in the Community) Act 1995. Current government announcements indicate the strong probability of the introduction of community treatment orders: '[Frank] Dobson confirmed this week that compulsory treatment [in the community] will be introduced for those posing the greatest threat to society' (*Community Care*, 10–16 December 1998, p.1). Indicative of the legal complexity of this issue however, is the report in the following week's edition of *Community Care*, on the appeal of a man with a diagnosis of schizophrenia, Anthony Smith, against a decision by the Mental Health Review Tribunal. Although the Tribunal took the view that Mr Smith's disorder was of a 'low degree' the nature of his condition warranted detention because he relapsed very quickly when he stopped taking his medication: 'The court heard that the clause of the Mental HealthAct 1983 which allows a person to be detained if the "nature or degree" of their condition warrants it, is generally ignored' (*Community Care*, p.1). *Community Care* comment that this confirms an opinion provided by Mental Health Act Commissioner Anselm Eldergill. Eldergill argued that there are already sufficient powers contained in the 1983 Act to detain 'patients refusing medication if: the nature of their disorder makes relapse inevitable; if they are a risk to themselves or others when the disorder is not controlled; and if there is evidence their condition is beginning to deteriorate ... Eldergill told *Community Care* that the ruling effectively made redundant the need for compulsory treatment orders. "The judgement confirms that patients may be detained if the nature of their disorder warrants"'. (*Community Care, ibid.*) (*Community Care*, 17 December 1998–6 January 1999, issue number 1253, p.1).

Concluding comments

We have reviewed the legal aspects of section 135 of the Mental Health Act 1983, in relation to case material. We have tried to demonstrate some practical difficulties and considerations which can arise, if the provisions of the Act are to be administered with due regard to sensitivity, whilst addressing issues of care and control. Increasingly, approved social workers, community psychiatric nurses, consultant psychiatrists and GPs are called on to be in the 'front-line' in terms of who is to undertake the meaningful caring for people with mental health problems, when institutions are either non-existent or, where they do exist, are too full to allow any further admissions.

12 Developing a psychotherapeutic approach to approved social work

Introduction

In this chapter we shall try to explore an approach to working with risk in approved social work, based on principles originating in psychoanalytic psychotherapy. This is a comparatively neglected method of approach to approved social work. Some of the key themes from each area are compared and contrasted through the use of case material. The argument is put forward that, through insights and skills derived from psychoanalytic psychotherapy, approved social workers can experience an improvement in their capacity to function in their role. Some key responsibilities can be achieved, particularly in the implementation of therapeutic principles and the non-use of compulsory powers of admission. Such issues are central to the approved social worker's role of promoting civil liberty, helping service users in non-punitive or persecutory ways, whilst at the same time continuing to promote public safety – in the approved social worker's monitoring role – and last, but not least, a better use of scarce hospital inpatient resources! In more radical ways, psychotherapeutically-oriented approved social workers can make available therapeutic relationships to people who, for reasons of class, status and finance, would not otherwise be able to afford 'therapy' or 'counselling'.

The relationship between psychoanalytic psychotherapy and approved social work has so far been a neglected area of study. Writers on the former have tended to concentrate on what might be termed the more recognisable, or easily acknowledged, areas of psychotherapy either in private practice or in NHS services (Hinshelwood, 1994; Healy, 1994; Denman 1994). Writers on the latter have focused on the bureaucratic or legalistic roles which the approved social worker necessarily embodies (Sheppard, 1990; Barnes *et al.*,

1990). Even in journal articles on multidisciplinary services, social work – in particular in its guise as the approved social worker – does not rate a mention (see, for example, Nightingale and Scott, 1994). Indeed, Bateman (1995) gives the social worker just one mention! Exceptions have been Winnicott (1963) and Valentine (1994). Valentine's article, 'The Social Worker as Bad Object', predominantly concerned social work with children and was an attempt to use psychoanalytically informed ideas to explore the negative image of social workers in the eyes of the public and the media. Interestingly, it met with some positive criticism from colleagues (Thomas, 1994). One of the authors of the present text has tried to explore elsewhere why social workers may be their own worst enemies in demonstrating the value of the social work profession to their colleagues (Thompson, 1995). In this chapter we try to explore this theme in relation both to risk and psychotherapy.

Risk

We deal in Chapter 9 with the very particular risk factors which are associated with dangerousness, both to self and others. Here, when we refer to risk we are talking in a more general sense. The approved social worker works perpetually in an atmosphere of risk; it is, as it were, our 'bread and butter'. This is a risk derived from the fact that people will only be referred to an approved social worker at a point of crisis, where there is, by definition, a high level of risk. It has become almost common parlance to observe that the Chinese symbol for crisis is that of a turning point, where a situation can change to very good or very bad. In that sense, a decision about how to intervene to try to resolve a situation of risk can result in a better or worse situation for all concerned. Approved social workers encounter this kind of dilemma when operating under the Mental Health Act. They must at once be able to distinguish between 'risk, hazard and danger' (in the words of CCETSW's paper 19.19), whilst also be able to 'have a much wider and more substantial role than merely reacting to requests for admission to hospital or guardianship' (CCETSW, 1993a). Carson offers the following definition of risk: 'An opportunity to gain possible benefits where harms are also possible' (Carson, 1995). In working with risk, Carson breaks the subject down into such areas as 'Risk factors ... Risk assessment ... Risk procedure ... Risk policy ... Risk management ... Risk decision-making' (ibid.).

The approved social worker is personally liable for his or her actions when operating in that role, yet at the same time is a functionary and a representative of their local authority. These two functions can sometimes be in conflict; indeed, depending on one's perceptions of how best to help people in situations of crisis, the two functions may inevitably always be in some tension. In order to try to work out how such a tension might be resolved, or at least reduced, we will first consider in more detail the issues relating to approved social work.

Approved social work

Approved social work and the approved social worker designation were terms introduced by the Mental Health Act 1983. They represented a return to the specialist function of mental health social work, or psychiatric social work, which had been eroded, if not actually destroyed, by the reorganisation of social services in 1970 when the concept of the 'generic' social worker had been introduced. The drafters of the Mental Health Act seemed to recognise the need for specialist training and expertise on the part of social workers responsible for people with mental health problems. (Jones (1994) provides introductory notes to some of the debates in parliament during the progress of the Act through the House of Commons and House of Lords.)

In order to be eligible for training to become 'approved' under section 114 of this Act, social workers were required to have at least two years' post-qualification training, unless they could demonstrate significant previous experience of working with people with mental health problems. Subsequent training consisted of at least 60 days' assessed attendance on courses approved by the Central Council for Training and Education in Social Work, including practical work placements in psychiatric hospitals. On the satisfactory completion of training, an approved social worker (ASW) received a warrant from their local authority which gave them a number of duties and powers. An approved social worker's primary duty is to

> ... make an application for admission to hospital or a guardianship application in respect of a patient within the area of the local social services authority by which that officer is appointed in any case where he is satisfied that such an application ought to be made and is of the opinion, having regard to any wishes expressed by relatives of the patient or any other relevant circumstances, that it is necessary or proper for the application to be made by him. (Section 13 (1), Mental Health Act 1983)

Approved social workers are personally liable for their actions whilst carrying out their functions under the Act, and are therefore obliged to act according to their own personal judgement, not that of employers, medical practitioners or others who might be involved with the patient's welfare (Jones, 1994). As indicated above, however, the approved social worker's role should be considered as being of a wider nature than simply considering such applications (CCETSW, 1993a).

Section 115 of the Mental Health Act confers a power on the approved social worker to 'enter and inspect' a premises, other than a hospital, where a mentally ill person may be living if he or she has reasonable cause to suspect that the patient may not be receiving adequate care. This is not a power to force access although, if access is denied, the approved social worker may apply to a magistrates' court under section 135 for a warrant to enable access to be forced with police assistance. Section 129 makes it an offence to obstruct an approved social worker in the performance of his or her statutory duties. Section 138 confers on the approved social worker the powers of a police constable to retake a patient who is escaping from custody. Sections 137 and 13 (3) extend the powers of approved social workers to enable them to carry out their responsibilities outside the area of the social services authority for which they were appointed (for example, if a patient known to the approved social worker requires assistance in another social services or health district).

There are at least four elements in the approved social worker's role which are pertinent to our considerations in the context of psychotherapeutic approaches and possibilities. The first is the personal responsibility of the approved social worker. Although the approved social worker is an officer of the local authority fulfilling statutory, and sometimes bureaucratic, requirements – filling in forms and so on – the approved social worker's judgements and accountability are personal. The second element is the requirement laid down in statute for the approved social worker to investigate all opportunities that might exist to prevent compulsory admission to, and detention in, a psychiatric hospital. This could, and in my experience has, involved the provision of someone to whom the patient can talk – including a continuing relationship with the approved social worker. The third element is the capacity of the approved social worker to act outside the geographic area of their usual responsibility – in other words, the approved social worker can follow the patient in an enduring way. The fourth element is the specialist mental health training and experience which the approved social worker must necessarily have to obtain their warrant.

Before considering some case material, it might be helpful to consider the factors we describe above in relation to psychoanalytic psychotherapy.

Psychoanalytical psychotherapy

Psychoanalysis and psychotherapy are be no means coterminous. The division between the British Confederation of Psychotherapists (BCP) and the United Kingdom Council for Psychotherapy (UKCP) are evidence of this in terms of professional organisation. In terms of clinical practice, Freud enjoined analysts to suspend all feelings, curiosity and 'therapeutic ambition' (Freud, 1912: 119) in order to best assist the patient. This has been more recently recapitulated by Bion in his injunction to the psychoanalyst to practise without 'memory or desire' (Bion, 1967: 144). This is a model of disinterest worthy of the Buddhist 'neither this nor that', or the early German Christian mystic, Meister Eckhardt who stated that 'one thing is necessary and that is disinterest' (Eckhardt, p.82)! That which helps the patient in analysis is the containment represented and acted out in the consulting room and the consistency of the analytic relationship. That which helps the psychoanalyst is the experience of their own analysis. This is 'pure' psychoanalyis, as derived from Freud. However, Freud did not believe that individuals with psychoses were able to be analysed, primarily because of their inability to form transference neuroses. Later clinicians (Klein, 1930; Rosenfield, 1947) have come to adopt a different view, that some patients with psychotic illnesses can benefit from psychoanalytic psychotherapy, although they may require modifications to the analytic technique, often requiring more intervention and sometimes involving practical management (Winnicott, 1963).

Indeed, in Klein's and Winnicott's early references to such treatment, they each refer to 'psychotherapy', rather than 'psychoanalytic psychotherapy'. In the same way that the psychotherapy of the psychoses can involve a modification of the psychoanalytic technique, so the institutional settings within which psychotherapy can be applied may also be open to modification so as not to be limited to the clinical setting. I want to argue that it is in those areas of severe psychotic disturbance where the patient passes beyond the usual range of psychoanalytic treatment and enters the realm of psychiatry or the penal system, that the approved social worker can have a special function. If the approved social worker holds some psychotherapeutic awareness he or she might be able to assist the service user and their relatives to integrate the four elements referred to above, with an approach based on relational understanding. In the best cases this can result in a diversion from the need for compulsory hospitalisation. In the worst cases, it can help make the process of compulsory hospitalisation more understandable and less threatening to the service user and, where appropriate, to their family, carers or close ones.

We now go on to consider these points in the context of some extended case material.

Case example 1

This example begins by demonstrating the way in which an approved social worker must work according to his or her individual judgement, sometimes acting against the requirements of the institution by which he or she is employed. This judgement may be affected by a number of factors. Not least, in terms of the psychotherapeutic dimension, will be the countertransference, together with the potential for therapeutic change, in the individual and his or her community, which this example goes on to consider. A countertransference relationship will, almost by definition, originate between individuals. How this relationship is experienced and worked through will determine to what extent its effects will ripple out and affect the larger institution.

Z was referred by a number of sources: these included his neighbours, the locally elected ward councillors and staff members of a nearby day centre. As is often the case in such referrals, Z was not aware of the level of local concern. Neither was it clear that local people who were concerned had been in contact one with another, although this seemed at least a possibility. The content of the concern was that Z frightened his neighbours. He was a big man, and his neighbours were largely elderly. Furthermore, he was black and his neighbours were all white. It was alleged that Z shouted and screamed at all hours of day and night. He had been heard banging very loudly in his flat. He had once or twice banged on the doors of his neighbours and then run away.

Z's ward councillor inferred that Z must recently have been 'released' from 'one of those mental hospitals which have been closed', with inadequate care and needed help before he harmed either himself or someone else.

The bureaucratic pressure on the approved social worker to whom this referral was made was to, in some way – indeed in any way – remove the nuisance which Z presented. Indeed, following the initial referral, the approved social worker received urgent correspondence from both the social service director and the director of housing to 'do' something (the director of housing having become involved because Z had ceased to pay his rent). The approved social worker felt somewhat overawed by these pressures although, at the same time, was conscious of his need to act in accordance with the requirements of the Mental Health Act, in terms of independence of assessment. The respective directorates are subject to the bureaucratic and political pressures imposed by their organisation on the one hand, or by their employers, the locally elected council members, on the other. The approved social worker is clearly subject to the cascade of pressure from those sources, yet at the same time carries a burden imposed by the requirements of the Act, which have an additional frame of reference in the sense that this work is monitored by the Mental Health Act Commission, in the context of pressure to act with due regard to patient sensitivity, antidiscriminatory practice, and civil liberties.

The approved social worker duly visited Z. He found him at home, but rather dishevelled in appearance. A probing, but non-threatening and non-persecutory, assessment interview revealed that Z was troubled by voices in his head which frightened him. These voices claimed that an international conspiracy involving figures from classical mythology threatened Z's life, but that he was all right, provided he did not go to a certain part of town that he associated with conspiracy because of ideas of reference to do with the names of certain streets. To prove his point he produced from inside his flat a children's book of mythology, pointing to the words (which he could just barely read) as if the words on the printed page were concrete evidence of the veracity of his thoughts. Z admitted that he had been frightening his neighbours, and was aware also that his appearance of being 'big and black' was difficult for some people to accept. He assured the approved social worker that he had no intention of going to that dangerous part of town because he knew if he did, he would end up being 'sectioned'. The approved social worker wondered whether Z might want to visit his office to talk about some of the frightening thoughts and feelings which he had. Z readily accepted this offer. Had he not accepted, the approved social worker felt that a further assessment would have had to have been arranged, probably leading to compulsory hospitalisation.

The approved social worker later reported back his findings to the social services and housing directors. Both senior officers were concerned that some more decisive action should have been taken, to remove a source of complaint within the local community. The approved social worker tried to make sense of the somewhat baffling range of demands and emotions at work here by an initial examination of his countertransference responses to Z in their doorstep interview. By 'countertransference responses', we mean what the approved social worker felt because, in psychoanalytic terms, feelings are communications to the same degree as words.

Z was indeed an imposing presence. He was tall, with a muscular build. He had huge, boxer's hands. His head was shaven. There was an immediate impression of potential violence. He had come to the door, in the middle of the day, wearing nothing but a short bathrobe. This evoked something possibly sexual, given that one of Z's neighbours was female and had felt frightened for her physical safety (she had found Z 'staring' at her one day in a common area of the building). The scrappy bathrobe seemed to represent Z's barely adequate attempts to veil his disturbance and keep it to himself. When Z spoke he seemed quite deferential, even apologetic. It was as if he was aware of the effect that his presence inspired and aware too of the menace both in his past and in his mind at that point, the 'dangerous part of town' representing the psychotic part of his mind which needed to be kept remote and secure.

To have proceeded with a compulsory admission after Z had accepted the offer of help could, apart from being illegal under the Mental Health Act, have been understood by Z as a retaliatory and persecutory reaction, so the approved social worker defended his position to his managers. Z kept his office appointment and agreed to begin meeting the approved social worker for regular sessions in order to talk about the thoughts, feelings and experiences which frightened him. These also were adhered to and, on consulting with those members of the community who had previously complained, it was acknowledged that, as these sessions continued, the disruption previously caused by Z's shouting and banging died down.

Comment and outcome

There appeared to be a complex interaction of projective identification elements at work here. The public disturbance caused by Z mirrored the disturbance in Z's mind, stimulating a requirement for control. This anxiety found its way to the approved social worker who concomitantly experienced a splitting of his loyalty between his employers and his professionalism, in a similar way to how the present elements of Z's mind were split apart and fragmented.

Correspondingly, the elements of racism at work in the locality seemed to be acting as a group phenomenon of projective identification insofar as the group, represented by the local community, were evacuating its unwanted elements into Z so that the pressure on Z from his neighbours (as well as the experience of living in an area known for racist attacks) was evoking a sense of heightened persecutory anxiety and probability of psychotic behaviour. Hinshelwood (1989) has discussed some of these processes more closely in regard to groups operating in therapeutic communities.

Nevertheless, there were also sufficient elements of concern about the safety of members of the public to indicate the necessity for some kind of formal intervention. It was the fact that Z still seemed to retain sufficient self-control as to refrain from visiting the 'dangerous part of town' that indicated to the approved social worker that there were sufficient reasons to believe that Z had not yet reached the point where compulsory intervention was the only viable alternative to other forms of treatment. In the course of Z's sessions it emerged from Z that he had a forensic history although the details of this could not be located by the approved social worker because the psychiatric hospital where he had been detained had been closed.

The commencement of sessions with the approved social worker in order to talk, in loosely defined terms, 'about his thoughts and feelings' corresponded shortly afterwards with the cessation of Z's troublesome behaviour. Z's rent payments too, began to be made. This relationship with the approved social worker, which took place under close monitoring by the worker's management, but continued on the basis of the personal responsibility of the approved social worker to make all attempts to seek an alternative to hospital detention (MHA s.13 (2)), resulted in the creation of a therapeutic relationship for Z, as well as preventing a full-scale compulsory admission under the Mental Health Act, which could have been a difficult and dangerous experience for all concerned.

Sessions continued for several months. It emerged that Z was really quite concerned for his neighbours and absolutely aware of the effect that his actual behaviour had on them, as well as the effect of his perceived appearance – his size, and his colour in the context of the community's realistic concerns, intermingled with some aspects of racism. No doubt Z's concern was with his capacity for violence and aggression, which had originally led him to his first prison sentence. In relation to the approved social worker's countertransference response, this was plainly one of profound fear and apprehension at being called on to assess a man with an unknown history, but amid a public clamour about dangerousness, in the unstructured setting of the man's own council flat, which he acknowledged he had wrecked during one psychotic episode.

Indeed, such was Z's shame at the state of his flat, that he requested that the initial assessment interview took place on the balcony outside the flat, because he did not want the approved social worker to see it. It is not difficult to infer that the 'state of the flat' represented the state of Z's mind. Both his flat and his mind were in a state of fragmentation as a result of Z's envious and destructive impulses. Indeed, it emerged that the considerable noise on one occasion had been Z kicking in his television set because he wanted to stop the broadcast from controlling his mind. Z did not want the extent of his fragmentation witnessed at that point, rather in the same way that Steiner describes the turning of a blind eye to psychic truth. At this point, the approved social worker was torn between imposing the relatively easy solution of a rapid and enforced hospitalisation, as against trying to acknowledge Z's wish to commence a therapeutic relationship, albeit of a tentative nature. The decision not to proceed with psychiatric assessments, and possibly an application under the Mental Health Act, was based on Z's expression of interest in talking about his feelings rather than acting them out. The fact that Z kept subsequent appointments and the cessation of nocturnal disruption seemed to confirm the efficacy of the therapeutic approach in this instance. The clamour from the local community died down.

Case example 2

X was a young woman who had been admitted to the psychiatric hospital from prison. Her index offence had been the theft of a baby (the baby having been recovered unharmed). Little was known with any certainty of her background, or her relationship with her parents, and she was ascribed a diagnosis of paranoid schizophrenia. At this point, she was homeless and was taken up by the approved social worker in order to assist with her rehousing. As is often the case, the issue of 'rehousing' began to mean much more and, through the medium of practical assistance, the establishment of a therapeutic relationship was enabled to take place. As discussed in example 1, this was not psychotherapy of the psychoanalytic description but, rather, took the form of supportive work and occasional, often brief, meetings between the worker and client.

The worker tried to ensure that the client/patient did not feel intruded upon or invaded yet, as in the example of Z, sought to ensure that the client/patient had a safe and contained space of their own. A further part of the analytical task – that of feeding back to the patient some of their more destructive and persecuted/persecutory feelings through interpretative work – becomes more complex when managing people in psychotic states of mind, precisely because such interpretations are experienced literally or in concrete terms, which can evoke increased persecutory states of mind in people in sometimes fragile circumstances (for example, people living alone, in bed and breakfast accommodation as X came to be).

Temporary accommodation was found for X and, on one of his visits, the approved social worker was presented with 30 line drawings which X had made over the preceding few months. It then emerged that X had trained as an artist, but had done no work for some time. It was with some surprise that the approved social worker took custody of these drawings, which she had done 'just for him'. Indeed, some were of him, some of her, and some of other things – the pet dog she used to have, a ship at sea, a basket of flowers.

The approved social worker felt touched by these pictures, but did not know what to make of either the fact of them or their meaning in their relationship. He took this to a consultancy session with the clinic's consultant psycho-therapist, who dismissed them as 'rubbish' – an interpretation that dismayed and confused the approved social worker who accepted it superficially, but felt that there was more to both the comment and the pictures. From the approved social worker's perspective the pictures were an attempt by X to hold their relationship in her mind, to work on it and digest it. Furthermore, because at least one of the pictures appeared to represent X naked, the approved social worker also hypothesised that elements of an erotic trans-ference were dawning, which he felt he needed to be conscious of.

With regard to the jibe of 'rubbish', the approved social worker felt that this exemplified how difficult that institution found it to accept the contri-bution that social work might make. The degree to which the consultant psychotherapist was right and the degree to which this was yet another instance of how the social worker's role in general, and the approved social role in particular, is misunderstood and devalued, is open to conjecture. Neither social work nor psychotherapy are exact sciences. Practitioners in each profession just do the best they can, and hope that their attempts make a positive contribution in the lives of the objects of their helpful intentions.

However, the best case that can be made for the comment and its effect on the social worker was that it created some confusion in in his mind, this muddle of not knowing what was rubbish and what was worthwhile, being, in turn, an unconscious communication arising through projective identification in the transference relationship between the social worker and his client.

Eventually, permanent accommodation was found for X in another area of the city and, with her agreement, social care was transferred to the local social work team for that area.

Some years passed, and one day the approved social worker received a duty call for X who had returned to his area of responsibility and required an assessment under the Mental Health Act. She was presenting a frightening and disruptive presence for her local community. She hoarded rubbish. She caused fires in the street. She fought with strangers in the street late at night. The approved social worker visited X, and she seemed to remember him. Although she was friendly enough to him, and put up no resistance, she was deluded and in need of psychiatric treatment, so the approved social worker arranged the appropriate medical examinations and tried to secure admission. At this point, X became hostile and tried to flee, having to be restrained by the approved social worker and then the police. Once in hospital, X made a relatively fast recovery, and was discharged to aftercare after a few weeks.

It will be noted that the theme of 'rubbish' arose again in the form of X's hoarding. The hoarding of rubbish is a common phenomenon in schizophrenia, and seems to represent the kind of muddle referred to above – of not being able to differentiate between what is ultimately good or bad, made manifest and concrete in a psychotic person's living situation. Sometimes the home of a schizophrenic can be completely taken over by an array of strangers, who wander in and out and represent the indigestible thoughts and feeling that the schizophrenic does not know what to do with. This can lead to an actual danger to the schizophrenic's safety, since some of those people may well have profound difficulties of their own.

Comment and outcome

The approved social worker kept X's pictures in his office, despite changing his office location a number of times. He did this for several reasons. The first reason was that he was never sure what they represented (in other words, they represented the 'muddle'). Second, he always felt that they were X's pictures, not his, and that he was their 'custodian', as in Winnicott (1963: 227): X's pictures were her eggs, and the approved social worker was the basket in Winnicott's terms. Third, he liked them and was touched by them. Fourth, he felt that, at some unknown point in the future, he might have some purpose for them, connected with X's future. In closing and transferring X's care initially, the worker was following correct departmental procedures, although there was perhaps also some unconscious relief at not having to contend with the unconscious muddle of their relationship, particularly in the area of the unresolved erotic transference. Thus, the pictures lay in his drawer like an unresolved series of communications residing in his mind.

An argument of this chapter is that it was in part the restitution of the relationship between client and worker or, more particularly, the remembering on the part of the worker, which enabled the client to make a rather better recovery from her severe illness than had taken place in the past. Another factor was that the social worker was able to rapidly assess X's needs and ensure compulsory hospitalisation at an early stage in her relapse, whereas previously she had needed to steal a baby in order to have her needs noticed – in other words, to be identified as an 'infant' who needed to be cared for.

Case example 3

The importance of remembering on the part of the approved social worker can be demonstrated in the example of W, a man with a recurring manic depressive illness of a bipolar type. The approved social worker had been allocated when W was an inpatient suffering a severe depressive episode. So serious had been that episode that W had neglected himself to the point of emaciation. Indeed, his teeth had begun to loosen and fall out and, at one point, it was feared that he would die during that admission. We might be reminded here of Freud and Klein's discussions of anxieties pertaining to biting, devouring or being devoured and the relationship to depressive anxiety (Freud, 1918; Klein, 1950). In fact, W recovered and returned to live alone in the community.

As is often the case, an ongoing relationship with the formal psychiatric services was terminated by W when he felt better. He saw no reason to continue any form of treatment.

Some years passed, during which time the approved social worker would occasionally bump into W in the street. Each acknowledged the meeting, the worker with a 'How are you?', the client with a 'Very well thank you'. W seemed to want no more involvement than that, and the worker respected W's apparent preference for non-involvement. There is, it seems, a balance between involvement and non-involvement in this work, correlating to Winnicott's description of the infant's need for space in order to achieve separation. A more formal need for involvement occurred one day when, by coincidence, the approved social worker in this case was on duty for emergency referrals and W was brought into the casualty unit by the police under a section 136.*

W had been picked up wandering down the middle of the main road, shouting incoherently. By the time the approved social worker had arrived to talk to W, he had begun to dismantle the hospital's electrical system. He seemed very agitated and restless, wore no shoes, and was of a dishevelled and unkempt appearance. On seeing the approved social worker, however, W instantly broke into a smile, sat down and stopped fiddling with the electrical wires on the wall (he had thought that the wires were connected to a secret surveillance system).

The approved social worker asked W what had been going on, as he seemed very troubled. W was able to explain that a relationship with a woman whom he cared about had broken up. He said he felt desperate. He said that he could only remember rushing out of the house to get help. The approved social worker explained that W had been brought to the hospital by the police, and that he and the doctors needed to decide what should happen next. Might W want to go into hospital? W said that he would very much like admission to hospital as a 'place of safety'. Consequently, in discussion with the duty psychiatrist, it was agreed to try a voluntary admission, but the approved social worker agreed to monitor events closely, in case W's consent proved too inconsistent, in which case considerations of the use of compulsory powers would have to be renewed – although this wasn't used as a lever to cajole W (the threat of legal sanction is expressly forbidden in the Act).

Comment and outcome

If the approved social worker who knew and had a relationship with W had not been available, it is probable from W's presentation that he would have been admitted to hospital under compulsion because, out of context, his behaviour and affect would have seemed most bizarre. Indeed, the duty psychiatrist and the approved social worker were themselves in two minds about which course of action was preferable. They both agreed on an informal admission, and the fact that this did not lead to formal powers becoming necessary on that admission might indicate the value of a sustained relationship between worker and client over a period of years, even at a low-key level. Indeed the work of Leff and Vaughan (1985) on expressed emotion would indicate that the balance between involvement and distance is crucial.

---

*Section 136 is a power residing with the police under the Mental Health Act to remove to a place of safety a person found in a public place who appears to be suffering from a mental disorder. Such an individual may be held for up to 72 hours in order for an assessment to be made by a doctor and an approved social worker.

In this case, W did remain committed to staying in hospital voluntarily and no formal application of the Act was necessary. This example also demonstrates, therefore, the way in which the persistence of the therapeutic relationships can assist in the important aspect of the approved social worker's role – that of seeking 'alternatives' to compulsory detention. Both the duty psychiatrist and duty approved social worker were agreed that this was the best way to manage W's admission on this occasion; however, at other times, W had been placed under a formal Mental Health Act order so that the section powers themselves would act as the containing environment and structure to replace the internal lack of structure and existence of chaos in W's mind.

In this context, W's perspective of the hospital as a 'place of safety' seems to me to be of interest and relevance if we compare this legal definition of a place that is deemed to be in some way 'safe' (because of the presence of caring nurses and doctors and so on, as well as the recourse to secure conditions if necessary) with the concept of an emotional safe place as found in the writings of Winnicott, Klein and Bion – particularly perhaps in the use of Bion's concept of the container and the contained. This can be particularly evinced in the personal, caring role of nursing staff as highlighted by Conran (1988, personal communication).

Conclusions

Compulsory admission to hospital is usually a frightening experience for service users; it is often traumatic for approved social workers too, if they have any sensitivity. Service users, as defined by the Mental Health Act 1983, automatically become 'patients' – a description which many people resent and would not wish to adopt; hence the preference for psychiatric service users to describe themselves as 'survivors' (Hastings and Crepaz-Keay, 1995). Survivors can feel stripped of rights and self-respect. Removing a person's freedom, either physically, as in their liberty, or metaphorically, in their freedom to decide on their lives and treatment choices, is a serious step.

We have tried to demonstrate that, by combining skills and insights derived from psychoanalytic psychotherapy, the approved social worker can assist some patients in obtaining psychiatric help without recourse to compulsion or the loss of liberty.

The approved social worker can use such skills to manage risk in positive ways. Where formal help within the terms defined by the Mental Health Act proves necessary, such skills can be applied to mitigate some of the worst effects experienced by long-term hospitalisation, and indeed seems, in some instances, to allow the promise of shorter periods of detention and faster remission. In our experience, many service users are actually relieved when the control which they have relinquished over their lives is removed from their responsibility, and an external containment, in the form of a 'section' is applied. (One person who ran away during the process assessment, when finally caught up with, promptly thanked the approved social worker for placing him under 'section'!) The Act conveys the authority to an approved social worker to assist in the specific restitution of a safe place in the lives of psychotic individuals. The powers and duties of the Act imply that this safe place is located externally. Through adequate understanding, sensitivity and partnership, safety can sometimes be achieved internally, through the creation of a safe, yet internal, emotional space for the service user.

Approved social workers often work with service users and in situations where inadequate understanding easily occurs. Such misunderstandings can arise on the part of our medical and nursing colleagues, not to say our clients, our patients and ourselves. These misunderstandings can be part of the splitting and attacking mechanisms connected with the psychotic process, acted out in institutions, or between professionals who are jointly engaged in the caring task. This final chapter has been one step in attempting a clarification of the approved social worker's position in these difficult and complex areas.

Appendix A: compulsory admission flowchart

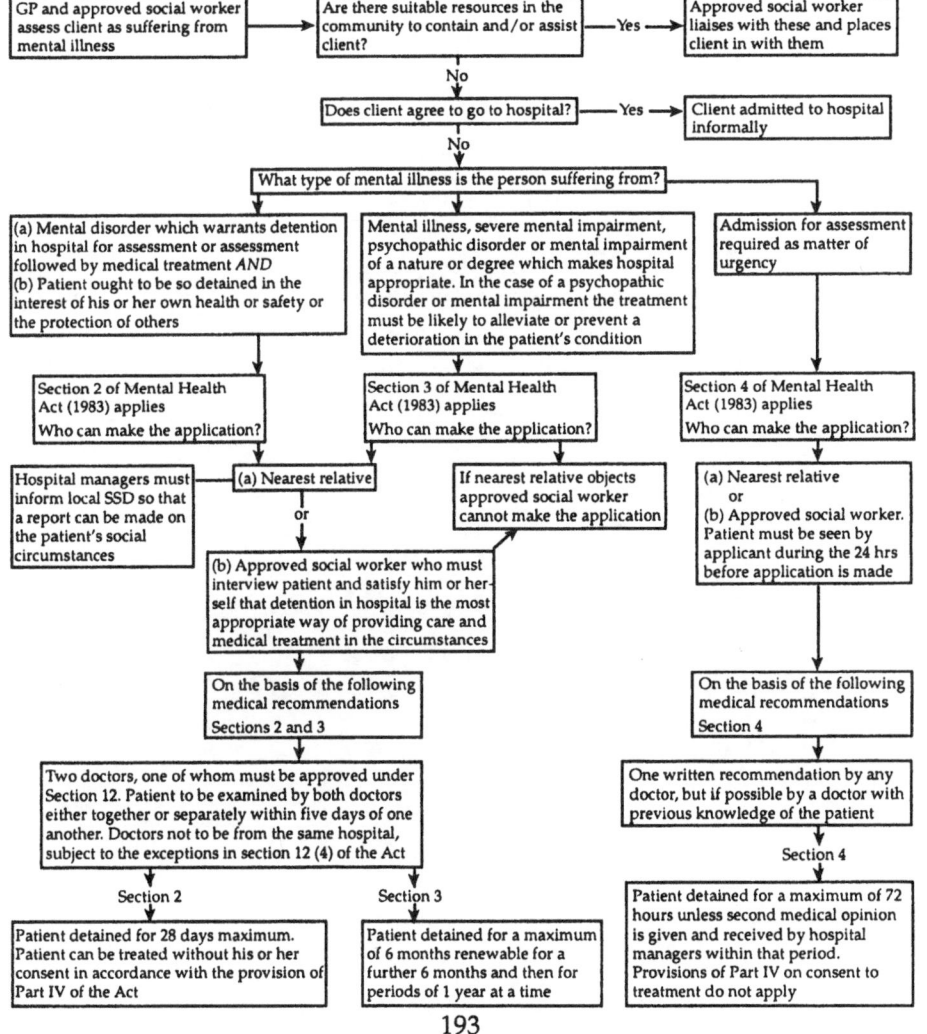

GP and approved social worker assess client as suffering from mental illness → Are there suitable resources in the community to contain and/or assist client? —Yes→ Approved social worker liaises with these and places client in with them

No ↓

Does client agree to go to hospital? —Yes→ Client admitted to hospital informally

No ↓

What type of mental illness is the person suffering from?

(a) Mental disorder which warrants detention in hospital for assessment or assessment followed by medical treatment *AND* (b) Patient ought to be so detained in the interest of his or her own health or safety or the protection of others

Mental illness, severe mental impairment, psychopathic disorder or mental impairment of a nature or degree which makes hospital appropriate. In the case of a psychopathic disorder or mental impairment the treatment must be likely to alleviate or prevent a deterioration in the patient's condition

Admission for assessment required as matter of urgency

Section 2 of Mental Health Act (1983) applies
Who can make the application?

Section 3 of Mental Health Act (1983) applies
Who can make the application?

Section 4 of Mental Health Act (1983) applies
Who can make the application?

Hospital managers must inform local SSD so that a report can be made on the patient's social circumstances

(a) Nearest relative
or

If nearest relative objects approved social worker cannot make the application

(a) Nearest relative
or
(b) Approved social worker. Patient must be seen by applicant during the 24 hrs before application is made

(b) Approved social worker who must interview patient and satisfy him or herself that detention in hospital is the most appropriate way of providing care and medical treatment in the circumstances

On the basis of the following medical recommendations
Sections 2 and 3

On the basis of the following medical recommendations
Section 4

Two doctors, one of whom must be approved under Section 12. Patient to be examined by both doctors either together or separately within five days of one another. Doctors not to be from the same hospital, subject to the exceptions in section 12 (4) of the Act

One written recommendation by any doctor, but if possible by a doctor with previous knowledge of the patient

Section 4

Section 2

Section 3

Patient detained for 28 days maximum. Patient can be treated without his or her consent in accordance with the provision of Part IV of the Act

Patient detained for a maximum of 6 months renewable for a further 6 months and then for periods of 1 year at a time

Patient detained for a maximum of 72 hours unless second medical opinion is given and received by hospital managers within that period. Provisions of Part IV on consent to treatment do not apply

Appendix B: statutory instruments

Children Act 1989

Data Protection Act 1984

DHSS No. LAC (86) 15: Approved Social Workers

Health and Safety at Work Act 1974

Housing Act 1985

Infanticide Act 1922 (amended 1938)

Local Government (Access to Information) Act 1985

Mental Health Act 1983

Mental Health (Patients in the Community) Act 1995

NHS and Community Care Act 1990

National Assistance Act 1948

Reporting of Injuries, Diseases and Dangerous Occurrences Regulations (RIDDOR) 1995

Police and Criminal Evidence Act 1984

References and further reading

Ahmed, S. (1993), *Practising Social Work*, ed. C. Hanvey and T. Philpot, London: Routledge.

Alcoholics Anonymous, *12 Steps*.

Atkinson, J.M. (1996), 'The Community of Strangers: Supervision and the New Right', *Health and Social Care in the Community*, 4 (2), 122–5.

Axiline, V. (1971), *Dibs in Search of Self*, Harmondsworth: Penguin.

Barnes, M., Bowl, R. and Fisher, M. (1990), *Sectioned*, London: Routledge.

Bateman, A. (1995), 'The Treatment of Borderline Patients in a Day Hospital Setting', *Journal of Psychoanalytic Psychotherapy*, 9 (1), 3–16.

Bateson, G. (1973), *Steps to an Ecology of Mind*, London: Paladin.

Bateson, G., Jackson, D., Haley, J. and Weakland, J. (1956), 'Towards a Theory of Schizophrenia, *Behavioural Science*, 1, 251.

Bhugra, D. (1997), *Psychiatry and Religion*, London: Routledge.

Bion, W.R. (1961), *Experiences in Groups*, London: Tavistock.

Bion, W.R. (1967), *Second Thoughts*, London: Heinemann.

Bion, W.R. (1977), *Seven Servants*, New York: Aaronson.

Blakney, R.B., Trans. (1941), *Meister Eckhardt*, New York: Harper & Row.

Brandon, D., Wells, K., Francis, C. and Ramsay, E. (1980), *The Survivors*, London: Routledge and Kegan Paul.

Breggin, P. (1993), *Toxic Psychiatry*, London: Harper Collins.

Brown, R., Bute, S. and Ford, P. (1988), *Social Workers at Risk*, London: Macmillan.

Brown, G.W., Carstairs, G.M. and Topping, G. (1958), 'Post-hospital adjustment of chronic mental patients', *Lancet II*, 655–9.

Carter, N., Klein, R. and Day, P. (1995), *How Organisations Measure Success*, London: Routledge.

Carson, D. (1995), 'Factors in risk assessment', *Community Care*, 26 October 1995.

CCETSW (1992), *Substance Use: Guidance notes for the DipSW*, London: CCETSW.

CCETSW (1993a), *Paper 19.19: Requirements and Guidance for the Training of Social Workers to be Considered for Approval in England and Wales Under the Mental Health Act 1983*, London: CCETSW.

CCETSW (1993b), *Paper 19.26: Approved Social Worker and Mental Health Officer Training*, London: CCETSW.

CCETSW (1993c), *Alcohol Problems*, ed. L. Harrison, London: CCETSW.

CCETSW (1993d), *Substance Misuse: Designing Social Work Training*, ed. I. Harrison, London: CCETSW.

CCETSW (1994), *Paper 19.29: Continuing Professional Education for Professional Social Workers*, ed. J. Jenkins and C. Whittington, London: CCETSW.

CCETSW (1995a), *Alcohol Interventions*, ed. R. Kemp, London: CCETSW.

CCETSW (1995b), *The Survivor's Guide to Training Approved Social Workers*, ed. M. Hastings and D. Crepaz-Keay, London:CCETSW.

Celan, P. (1980), *Collected Poems*, Carcanet.

Chasseguet-Smirgel, J. (1985), *Creativity and Perversion*, London: Free Association Books.

Craig, T., Bayliss, E., Klein, O., Manning, P. and Reader, L. (1995), *The Homeless Mentally Ill Initiative*, London: Department of Health/Mental Health Foundation.

Dalal, F. (1988), 'The Racism of Jung', *Race and Class*, **29** (3).

Dalton, K. (1982), 'Legal Implications of PMS', *World Medicine*, **17**, 93–4.

Davies, M. (1994), *The Essential Social Worker*, Aldershot: Arena.

Denman, F. (1994), 'The Value of Psychotherapy', *British Journal of Psychotherapy*, **11** (2), Winter.

Department of Health (1996), *Statistical Bulletin 1996/10*, June, London: HMSO.

De Shazer, S. (1985), *Keys to Solution in Brief Therapy*, New York: W.W. Norton.

d'Orban, P.T. (1983), 'Medico-Legal Aspects of the Pre-Menstrual Syndrome', *British Journal of Hospital Medicine*, **30**, 404–9.

Eliade, M. (1964), *Shamanism*, New York: Bollingen.

Erikson, E. (1965), *Childhood and Society*, Harmondsworth: Penguin.

Everyone's Guide to Riddor (1995), London: HSE Books.

Fennell, P. (1989), 'The Beverley Lewis case: was the law to blame?', *New Law Journal*, November 17, 1557–8.

Fernando, S. (1991), *Mental Health, Race and Culture*, London: Macmillan/MIND.

Fernando, S. (1995), *Mental Health in a Multi-Ethnic Society*, London: Routledge.

Fernando, S., Ndegwa, D. and Wilson, M. (1998), *Forensic Psychiatry, Race and Culture*, London: Routledge.

Fisher, K. and Collins, J. (1993), *Homelessness, Health Care and Welfare Provision*, London: Routledge.

Fordham, M. (1995), *The Fenceless Field*, London: Routledge.

Fordham, M., Gordon, R., Hubback, J. and Lambert, K. (eds) (1979), *Technique in Jungian Analysis*, London: Heinemann.

Foulkes, S.H. (1964), *Therapeutic Group Analysis*, London: Allen and Unwin.

Foulkes, S.H. (1975), *Group Analytic Psychotherapy*, London: Gordon and Branch.

Freud, S. (1905), *Three Essays on the Theory of Sexuality*, standard edn, Vol. 6, London: Hogarth Press.

Freud, S. (1912), *Recommendations to Physicians Practising Psychoanalysis*, standard edn, Vol. 12, London: Hogarth Press.

Freud, S. (1913), *Totem and Taboo*, standard edn, Vol. 13, London: Hogarth Press.

Freud, S. (1917), *Introductory Lectures*, standard edn, Vol. 16, London: Hogarth Press.

Freud, S. (1918), 'From the History of an Infantile Neurosis', in *The Standard Edition of the Complete Psychological Works*, Vol. XVII, London: Hogarth Press.

Freud, S. (1930), *Civilization and its Discontents*, standard edn, Vol. 21, London: Hogarth Press.

Freud S. (1975), Group Psychology and the Analysis of the Ego, standard edn of S. Freud, Vol. 18, London: Hogarth Press.

Fromm, E. (1974), *The Anatomy of Human Destructiveness*, London: Cape.

Frosch, S. (1989), 'Psychoanalysis and Racism', in B. Richards (ed.), *Crises of the Self*, London: Free Association Books.

Gaarder, J. (1996), *Sophie's World*, London: Orion Books.

Gandhi, M.K. (1927), *An Autobiography*, Ahmedabad: Navajivan Publishing House.

George, E., Iveson, C. and Ratner, H. (1990), *Problem to Solution: Brief Therapy with Individuals and Families*, London: Brief Therapy Press.

Goldberg, D. and Huxley, P. (1980), *Mental Illness in the Community*, London: Tavistock.

Gordon, P. (1993), 'Souls in Armour: Thoughts on Psychoanalysis and Racism', *British Journal of Psychotherapy*, **10** (1), 62–77.

Hafner, H. and Boker, W. (1973), *Crimes of Violence by Mentally Disordered Offenders. A psychiatric and epidemiological study in the Federal German Republic* (trans. H. Marshall, 1982).

Hall, S. and Jefferson, T. (1975), *Resistance through Rituals*, London: Hutchinson.

Hastings, M. and Crepaz-Keay, D. (1995), *A Survivor's Guide to ASW Training*, London: CCETSW.

Healy, K. (1994), 'Why Purchase Psychotherapy Services?', *British Journal of Psychotherapy*, **11** (2), 279–84.

Hillman, J. (1995), *Kinds of Power*, New York: Doubleday.

Hinshelwood, R.D. (1987), *What Happens in Groups*, London: Free Association Books.

Hinshelwood, R.D. (1989), *A Dictionary of Kleinian Thought*, London: Free Association Books.

Hinshelwood, R.D. (1994), 'The Relevance of Psychotherapy', *Psychoanalytic Psychotherapy*, **8** (3), 283–94.

HMSO (1991), *Disasters: Planning for a Caring Response*, London: HMSO.

HMSO (1995), *Volatile Substance Abuse: A Report by the Advisory Council on the Misuse of Drugs*, London: HMSO.

Hoggett, B. (1996), *Mental Health Law*, 4th edn, London: Sweet and Maxwell.

Howe, D. (1996), 'Surface and depth in social work practice', in N. Parton (ed.), *Social Theory, Social Change and Social Work*, London: Routledge.

Hudson, B. (1982), *Social Work with Psychiatric Patients*, London: Allen and Unwin.

Huxley, P. and Kerfoot, M. (1993), 'The Mental Health Workforce in the Community', *Health and Social Care*, **1**, 169–74.

Huxley, P. and Kerfoot, M. (1994), 'A Survey of Approved Social Work in England and Wales', *British Journal of Social Work*, **24**, 311–24.

Illich, I. (1977), *Disabling Professions*, London: Marion Boyars.

Jacques, E. (1970), *Work, Creativity and Social Justice*, London: Heinemann.

Jenkins, R. *et al.* (1994), *The Prevention of Suicide*, London: HMSO.

Jones, E. (1977), *The Life and Work of Sigmund Freud*, Harmondsworth: Pelican.

Jones, R. (1996), *Mental Health Act Manual*, 5th edn, London: Sweet and Maxwell.

Jung, C.G. (1911, reprinted 1956), *Collected Works*, Vol. 5, London: Routledge and Kegan Paul.

Jung, C.G. (1918), 'The Role of the Unconscious', *Collected Works*, Vol. 10, London: Routledge and Kegan Paul.

Jung, C.G. (1930), 'The Complications of American Psychology', *Collected Works*, Vol. 10, London: Routledge and Kegan Paul.

Jung, C.G. (1936), 'Yoga and the West', *Collected Works*, Vol. 11, London: Routledge and Kegan Paul.

Jung, C.G. (1939a), 'What India Can Teach Us', *Collected Works*, Vol. 10, London: Routledge and Kegan Paul.

Jung, C.G. (1939b), 'Foreword to Suzuki's "Introduction to Zen Buddhism"', *Collected Works*, Vol. 11, London: Routledge and Kegan Paul.

Jung, C.G. (1950), *Collected Works*, Vol. 9, Part 2, London: Routledge and Kegan Paul.

Jung, C.G. (1954), 'Psychological Commentary on the "Tibetan Book of the Great Liberation"', *Collected Works*, Vol. 11, London: Routledge and Kegan Paul.

Jung, C.G. (1955), *Collected Letters*, Vol. 2, London: Routledge and Kegan Paul.

Jung, C.G. (1963a), 'Mysterium Coniunctonis', *Collected Works*, Vol. 14, London, Routledge and Kegan Paul.

Jung, C.G. (1963b), 'Memories, Dreams and Reflection', London: Routledge and Kegan Paul.

Jung, C.G. (1968), 'The Archetypes and the Collective Unconscious', *Collected Works*, Vol. 9, Part 1, London: Routledge and Kegan Paul.

Jung C.G. (1976), 'The Practice of Psychotherapy', *Collected Works*, Vol. 16, London: Routledge and Kegan Paul.

Kernberg, O. (1975), *Borderline Conditions and Pathological Narcissism*, New York: Aronson.

Kernberg, O. (1993), *Severe Personality Disorders*, New Haven, Conn.: Yale University Press.

Kahn, J. (1971), *Human Growth and the Development of Personality*, Oxford: Pergamon.

Kearney, B. (1989), 'Mad, Bad and Dangerous to Know', in C. Rojek, G. Peacock and S. Collins (eds), *The Haunt of Misery*, London: Routledge.

King, M., Coker, E., Leavey, G., Hoare, A. and Johnson-Sabine, E. (1994), 'Incidence of Psychotic Illness in London: A Comparison of Ethnic Groups', *British Medical Journal*, **309** (6962), 29 October.

Klein, M. (1929), 'Love, Guilt and Reparation', in *The Writings of Melanie Klein*, Vol. I, London: Hogarth Press (1975).

Klein, M. (1930), 'The Psychotherapy of the Psychoses', in *Love, Guilt and Reparation and Other Works 1921–1945*, London: Hogarth Press.

Klein M. (1946), 'Notes on Some Schizoid Mechanisms', in *The Writings of Melanie Klein*, Vol. III, London: Hogarth Press (1980).

Klein, M. (1950), 'On the Criteria for the Termination of Psycho-Analysis', in *Envy and Gratitude and Other Works 1946–1963*, London: Hogarth Press (1980).

Klein, M. (1957), 'Envy and Gratitude', in *The Writings of Melanie Klein*, Vol. III, London: Hogarth Press (1980).

Kuipers, L., McCarthy, B., Hurry, J. and Harper, R. (1989), 'Counselling the Relatives of the Long Stay Adult Mentally Ill', *British Journal of Psychiatry*, **154**, 775–82.

Laing, R.D. (1960), *The Divided Self*, London, Tavistock.

Laing, R.D. (1973), *Knots*, London: Penguin.

Laing, R.D. and Esterson, A. (1966), *Sanity, Madness and the Family*, Harmondsworth: Penguin.

Laplanche, J. and Pontalis, J.B. (1973), *The Language of Psychoanalysis*, London: Hogarth Press.

Laufer, M. (1975), *Adolescent Disturbance and Breakdown*, Harmondsworth: Penguin.

Leech, K. (1975), *Youthquake*, London: Sheldon Press.

Leff, J. (1997), *Care in the Community – Illusion or Reality?*, Chichester: Wiley.

Leff, J. and Vaughn, C. (1980), 'The Interaction of Life Events and Relatives'

Expressed Emotion in Schizophrenia and Depressive Neurosis', *British Journal of Psychiatry*, **136**, 146–53.

Leff, J. and Vaughn, C.E. (1985), *Expressed Emotion in Families: Its Significance for Mental Illness*, London: Guildford Press.

Lipstadt, D. (1994), *Denying the Holocaust*, Harmondsworth: Penguin.

Lowe, P. and Lewis, R. (1994), *Management Development Beyond the Fringe*, London: Kogan Page.

Lucas, R. (1994), 'Puerperal Psychosis: Vulnerability and Aftermath', *Psychoanalytic Psychotherapy*, **8** (3), 257–72.

McCall, K. (1982), *Healing the Family Tree*, London: Sheldon Press.

Mann, S.A. and Cree, W. (1976), 'New Long Stay Psychiatric Patients: A National Sample Survey of Fifteen Mental Hospitals in England and Wales 1972/3', *Psychological Medicine*, **6**, 603–16.

Masson, J. (1984), *Freud – The Assault on Truth*, Boston: Faber and Faber.

Matthews, C. (1991), *Sophia – Goddess of Wisdom*, London: Mandala Books.

Mayberry, J.F. (1996), 'Views of Professionals and Patients on Compulsory Removal from Home to an Institution', *Health and Social Care*, **4** (4), 208–14.

Mental Health Act Commission (1995), *Sixth Biennial Report 1993–5*, London: HMSO.

Menzies-Lyth, I. (1988), *Containing Anxiety in Institutions*, London: Free Association Books.

Menzies-Lyth, I. (1989), *The Dynamics of the Social*, London: Free Association Books.

Minuchin, S. (1974), *Families and Family Therapy*, Cambridge, Mass.: Harvard University Press.

Naik, D. (1992), 'The Politics of Anti-racist Requirements and the Role of the External Assessor in Relation to Programmes and Programme Providers', *Issues in Social Work Education*.

Nightingale, A. and Scott, D. (1994), 'Problems of Identity in Multi-disciplinary Teams', *British Journal of Psychotherapy*, **11** (2).

Norris, D. (1990), *Violence Against Social Workers*, London: Jessica Kingsley.

North, M. (1972), *The Secular Priests*, London: George Allen and Unwin.

Nottingham Community Health NHS Trust and Nottingham Community Drug Prevention Team (1994), *Focus Drug Information Booklet*.

Obholzer, A. and Roberts, V.Z. (1995), *The Unconscious at Work*, London, Routledge.

O'Hagan, K. (1986), *Crisis Intervention in Social Services*, London: Macmillan.

O'Hagan, K. (1994), *Practising Social Work*, London: Routledge.

Payne, M. (1991), *Modern Social Work Theory*, London: Macmillan.

Peterson, D. (1982), *A Mad People's History of Madness*, Pittsburg: University of Pittsburg Press.

Philpot, T. and Hanvey, C. (1994), *Practising Social Work*, London: Routledge.

Piaget, J. (1953), *The Origin of Intelligence in the Child*, London: Routledge and Kegan Paul.

Pietroni, M. (1995), 'The Nature and Aims of Professional Education for Social Workers', in M. Yelloly and M. Henkel (eds), *Learning and Teaching in Social Work*, London: Jessica Kingsley.

Prins, H. (1995), *Offenders, Deviants or Patients*, London: Routledge.

Prior, P. (1992), 'The Approved Social Worker – Reflections on Origins', *British Journal of Social Work*, **22**, 105–19.

Reder, P., Duncan, S. and Gray, M. (1993), *Beyond Blame*, London: Routledge.

Report of Confidential Inquiry into Homicides and Suicides by Mentally Ill People (1996), London: Royal College of Psychiatrists.

Richards, B. (1989), *Crises of the Self*, London: Free Association Books.

Richards, B. (1995), *Disciplines of Delight*, London: Free Association Books.

Richie, J.H. (1994), *The Report of the Inquiry into the Care and Treatment of Christopher Clunis*, London: HMSO.

Rojek, C., Peacock, G. and Collins, S. (1988), *Social Work and Received Ideas*, London: Routledge.

Rojek, C., Peacock, G. and Collins, S. (1989), *The Haunt of Misery*, London: Routledge.

Rosenfield, H.A. (1947), 'Analysis of a Schizophrenic State with Depersonalization', in *Psychotic States: A Psychoanalytic Approach*, London: Karnac Books (1982).

Rosenfield, H. (1964), *Psychotic States*, London: Maresfield Reprints (1984).

Rustin, M. (1991), *The Good Society and the Inner World*, London: Verso Books.

Rutter, M. (1974), *Helping Troubled Children*, Harmondsworth: Penguin.

Rutter, M. (1981), *Maternal Deprivation Reassessed*, 2nd edn, Harmondsworth: Penguin.

Rutter, M. and Gould, M. (1985), 'Classification', in M. Rutter and L. Hersov (eds), *Child and Adolescent Psychiatry: modern approaches*, 2nd edn, London: Blackwell.

Samuels, A. (1989), *Psychopathology: Contemporary Jungian Perspectives*, London: Karnac.

Samuels, A. (1993), *The Political Psyche*, London: Routledge.

Satir, V. (1964), *Conjoint Family Therapy*, Palo Alto: Science and Behaviour Books.

Schneider, K. (1959), *Clinical Psychopathology*, New York: Grune and Stratton.

Segal, H. (1981), *Introduction to the Work of Melanie Klein*, London: Hogarth Press.

Sheppard, D. (1991), 'Giving ASWs the Back-up They Need', *Community Care*, 28 November.

Sheppard, M. (1990), *Mental Health: The Role of the Approved Social Worker*, London: Joint Unit for Social Services Research/Community Care.

Sheppard, M. (1991), 'Walking the Tightrope', *Community Care*, 28 November.

Sinason, V. (1991), *Satanic Abuse*, London: Routledge.

Sinason, V. (1994), *Mental Handicap and the Human Condition*, London: Routledge.

Singer, J. (1977), *Androgyny*, London: Routledge and Kegan Paul.

Skinner, B.F. (1953), *Science and Human Behaviour*, New York: Macmillan.

Skynner, A.C.R. (1976), *One Flesh, Separate Persons – Principles of Family and Marital Psychotherapy*, London: Constable.

Spokes Report into the Murder of Isobel Schwarz (1987), London: HMSO.

Steiner, J. (1982), 'Personal Psychotherapy in the Training of a Psychiatrist', *Bulletin of the Royal College of Psychiatrists*, March, 41.

Steiner, J. (1983), 'Turning a Blind Eye to Oedipus', lecture given to staff of Friern Hospital.

Thomas, N. (1994), 'The Social Worker as Bad Object: A Response to M. Valentine', *British Journal of Social Work*, 24 (6), December.

Thompson, P.J. (1995), 'New Directions in Social Services and Education', *Practice – A Journal of the British Association of Social Workers*, 7 (4).

Tyler, A. (1995), *Street Drugs*, London: Coronet.

Valentine, M. (1994), 'The Social Worker as Bad Object', *British Journal of Social Work*, 24 (1), February.

Valios, N. (1996), 'Report Says that Social Workers' Stress Levels are Rising', *Community Care*, 9–16 February.

Walsh, C. (1996), *Professional Social Work*, London: BASW.

Webb, D. (1996), in N. Parton (ed.), *Social Theory, Social Change and Social Work*, London: Routledge.

Wing, J.K. (1981), 'Asperger's Syndrome: a clinical account', *Psychological Medicine*, 11, 115–30.

Wing, J.K. and Brown, J. (1970), *Institutionalism and Schizophrenia*, Cambridge: Cambridge University Press.

Winnicott, D.W. (1947), 'Hate in the Counter-Transference', in *Through Paediatrics to Psycho-Analysis*, London: Hogarth Press (1982).

Winnicott, D.W. (1963), 'Psychotherapy of the Character Disorders' and 'The Mentally Ill in Your Caseload', in *The Maturational Processes and the Facilitating Environment*, London: Hogarth Press (1982).

Wolff, H., Bateman A. and Sturgeon, D. (eds) (1990), *UCH Textbook of Psychiatry*, London: Duckworth.

Wolpe, J. (1958), *Psychotherapy by Reciprocal Inhibition*, Stanford, Cal.: Stanford University Press.

Woodley Team Report (1995), London: East London and City Health Authority/Newham Council.

Zweig, S. (1949–51), *Kaleidescope 1/2*, London: Cassell Press.

Index